THE SPLEEN AND STOMACH

Monkey Press is named after the Monkey King in The Journey to the West, the 16th century classical novel by Wu Chengen. Monkey blends skill, initiative and wisdom with the spirit of freedom and irreverence.

Chinese Medicine from the Classics
Claude Larre and Elisabeth Rochat de la Vallée

The Heart in Lingshu chapter 8
The Secret Treatise of the Spiritual Orchid: Suwen chapter 8
The Lung
The Kidneys
The Liver
Spleen and Stomach
Heart Master, Triple Heater
The Way of Heaven: Suwen chapters 1 and 2

CHINESE MEDICINE FROM THE CLASSICS

Claude Larre and Elisabeth Rochat de la Vallée

THE SPLEEN AND STOMACH

A Monkey Press Publication

Published by
M o n k e y P r e s s
36 Richmond Road
Cambridge
CB4 3PU

CHINESE MEDICINE FROM THE CLASSICS: THE SPLEEN AND STOMACH
Claude Larre and Elisabeth Rochat de la Vallée
Reprinted 1996

ISBN 1 872468 03 9

Series Editor: Peter Firebrace
Text Editor: Caroline Root
Production and Design: Sandra Hill
Calligraphy: Qu Lei Lei

Cover design: Mark Jacobs
Calligraphy: *pi wei* by Qu Lei Lei

Printed on recycled paper by Spider Web, London

FOREWORD

As Chinese - or, more properly, Oriental - medicine evolves in the different schools, colleges and courses and through the constant practice of acupuncturists, herbalists, practitioners of *shiatsu, tui na, qi gong, tai ji* and the martial arts, source books are needed that present an unbiased view of its principles and foundation concepts, without leanings toward a particular line of end-thinking. By working directly from the original medical texts, no position is taken - other than that of the original seed authors themselves. This is the aim of the **Chinese Medicine from the Classics** series: to help establish that primary level of understanding which is central to every aspect of the subject, a firm foundation for development later into a specific line of thinking or way of working.

Claude Larre and Elisabeth Rochat de la Vallee, of the Ricci Institute and European School of Acupuncture in Paris, are both lecturers of international repute who have helped to preserve the vitality and depth of Chinese thought with their special blend of scholarship, perception and humour. They bring to Chinese medicine all the benefits of their long-term study of Chinese culture and thinking in general and their deep and detailed knowledge of the Daoist texts in particular, shedding light on what can, without guidance, seem obscure, abstruse or confused, giving the feel of the Chinese perspective as much as the actual words themselves.

The Lung and **The Kidneys** have already been published in this series - the master and the root of *qi,* the upper and lower source of water. This book covers the Spleen/Stomach and the next, the Heart, shifting the emphasis from above/below to different expressions of Centre. The Heart commands through the Void, all-clear Spirit channel, central to Heaven's circling rhythms; Spleen/Stomach the dynamic duo of stability through constant change, the central transformative power of Earth.

Ancient terms - *yun hua* transporting and transforming, *qing zhuo* clear and unclear - these are highly topical to the Earth 'outside' with our eleventh hour realisation of the delicate balanced chaining and interconnection of all life systems and species: the land, our Mother Earth, unable to transform the poisons spread on the fields, the rivers and seas unable to cleanse themselves of effluence, pollution, *zhuo* where there should be *qing*. But where where does all that begin? 'Inside', with a lack of nourishment and proper respect for our own body Earth, our fleshy substantial, personal Earth that itself connects to *si* , thinking, the clear or the unclear mind, the pure or the impure thought, eating away.

China - *zhong guo* - the Central Kingdom - has always had a special understanding of centre and being centred and we would be wise to take note of their insights into Earth in us with all its many resonances given in Su Wen Chapters 4 and 5. The painstaking work Elisabeth Rochat has made presenting references to the Spleen and Stomach in different contexts in the Nei Jing, so adding one facet here and another there, builds up to give an organic understanding of the process each represents and their many manifestations and interconnections.

Many thanks to Claude Larre and Elisabeth Rochat for the seminar itself and helping to check the written form; to Caroline Root for the transcribing and editing of the text; Sandra Hill for the co-ordination, layout and design and to Qu Lei Lei for the calligraphy throughout. Each has had an essential role to play in the book's production.

It is hoped that the book will act as a catalyst for the reader, stimulating new thought which in turn will enrich and enhance practice through whatever medium and whatever system.

Peter Firebrace
Series editor
London
September 1990

CONTENTS

Spleen/Stomach pathology

Illustrations

Cover
Background Design: Daoist talisman related to Heaven
from Zheng Tong Dao Zang
Calligraphy: Spleen and Stomach, *pi wei,* Qu Lei Lei

Frontispiece
The Daoist Yellow Book Talisman related to Earth
from Zheng Tong Dao Zang

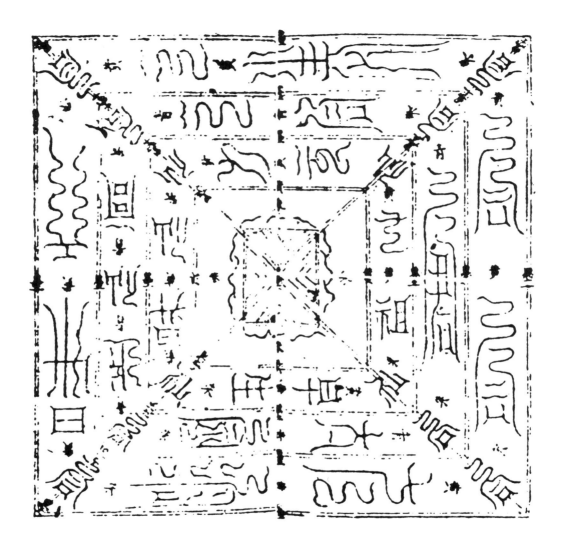

The Daoist Yellow Book talisman related to Earth

INTRODUCTION

Elisabeth Rochat: If we were to say that Stomach and Spleen act as a Centre, then we have said absolutely everything. But the important thing is to understand what the effect of this role of being a Centre is, and what sort of processes are implied in this English word. We will begin with the ideograms and through them and their analysis we can have the first idea of Spleen and Stomach in the Chinese language.

Claude Larre: When Elisabeth was talking of 'Centre', she could be talking of the same function as the Heart, because the Heart is the centre of life, but this is not at the same level. The Chinese say the Centre of life is the Stomach and Spleen, or they say that the Centre of life is the Heart. Or they say that the principle of life is the Kidneys, or they say that the extension of life is the Liver. All these terms, similar or dissimilar, are true at the same time but not from the same point of view.

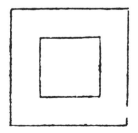

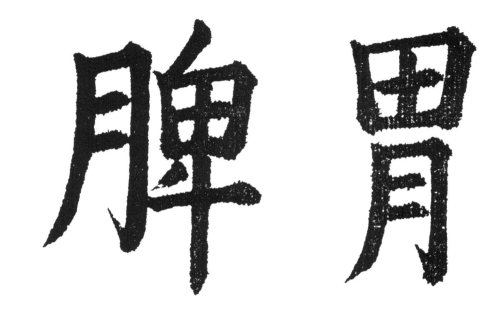

Pi Wei, Spleen and Stomach

The ideogram for the Spleen, *pi*

月
卑
尊

卑

府 藏

裨
婢
俾

Elisabeth Rochat: The ideogram for the Spleen has two parts - one is the radical, the flesh, which indicates that the ideogram designates part of the body, and the other is the graphic part which is etymologically an ancient drinking vessel, provided with a handle on the left side. This kind of vessel was used every day, for common activities, as opposed to another kind of vessel, *zun*, which was used uniquely for sacrifices. These two ideograms, which originally designated the vessel that was commonly used and the special vessel for sacrifices, give the meaning of ordinary, vulgar for the first common vessel, and honourable for the second vessel used for sacrifices.

In classical Chinese the ideogram *pi* has the meaning of ordinary or vulgar, just like this first vessel. We can see that the Spleen is really like a servant who works every day, all day and even on Sunday, and we'll see that too, with some of the correspondences with the Earth Element, and Spleen. For example, the ox, associated with the Earth Element, is an animal which works every day during all the year in order to cultivate the earth. We also see that the Spleen, as a kind of servant of the vitality, has a very common and ordinary task - but it is a task that is necessary for life. We see in a quotation from the Nei Jing that among the *zang* the Spleen is the nearest to the *fu*, which have to do with transportation, transformation and all these common, ordinary and quite vulgar tasks for the maintenance of vitality.

If we have another look at the ideogram with the same main graphic part (the phonetic) and we just change the radical to that of clothes instead of flesh, we have the ideogram with the meaning of to aid, to benefit, to be here in order to help somebody in his task. If we add the radical of woman we have the meaning of servant, slave girl, who in ancient times was in charge of grinding up the grain in the palace of the lords. If we just add the radical of human activity, we have an ideogram with the meaning of to enable, to cause, to act so that we do something. If you add the radical of disease (this is a slight transformation in the graphics, but the meaning is the same) this becomes a kind of disease, *bi*, that

3

you all know well: the type of blockage in circulation due to an exterior perverse attack of cold, humidity and wind. We also have some other kinds of ideograms with this radical, or with this phonetic and other radicals such as liquid or cereal or stalk giving the meaning of different kinds of rice or wheat or some kind of cereals.

So to summarize, we have the idea of something in the body which is always at work, like a slave girl, doing very obscure work, to help something very deeply, in order to bring forth something necessary, and to enable something to happen. I think that these are the main significations just from the ideograms.

The ideogram for the Stomach, *wei*

Elisabeth Rochat: The second ideogram is Stomach. You can see that we have the same radical, a part of the body, but it is not on the left side but on the lower part. Etymologically the top part is not the idea of the field, as you might imagine because although there is a similar Chinese ideogram with the meaning of a very well cultivated field it's not that. The etymological Chinese explanation is that this is some space, an area in which food is enclosed, and if you reverse this inner part of the upper character which is grain (Radical 119) you have the same graphic element as in the ideogram for Essences, *jing*. But that is just an additional remark. This is the Stomach, the part of the body, and the function in the body which encloses food in the shape of grains. It is said that in ancient times - it may be true or not - that this ideogram alone without the lower part, flesh, had the meaning of Stomach. It's like a sack, a pocket full of grains. It is very difficult to say anything else because the meaning is obvious. It's a receptacle for food, for grains, and it is also a typical example of a *fu,* a *fu* which is a receptacle, receiving food at its own level, in order to do something. We can remember these etymological explanations when we find that Spleen and Stomach have charge of granaries and storehouses.

SU WEN CHAPTER 8

The Spleen and Stomach as storehouses and granaries, *cang lin*

Spleen and Stomach are in charge of storehouses and granaries
The five tastes stem from them.

Elisabeth Rochat: We find these definitions of Spleen and Stomach for the first time in the Nei Jing in Su Wen Chapter 8. It's a very short quotation, but we have already had a full seminar on Chapter 8 of the Su Wen, in which the entire hierarchy of the twelve viscera was shown, with the Heart coming first, and afterwards Lung, Liver, Gall Bladder, *tan zhong*, and in the sixth position, Spleen and Stomach. And we can see why - because the centre is in the sixth position.

膻中

Claude Larre: Maybe for people who are not familiar with that chapter we should explain. There are eleven lines and the sixth line leaves five above and five below, so graphically speaking this line where Spleen and Stomach are put is really the axis around which all is revolving. In that sense to see the text, and to see that it is well disposed, gives you the impression of what the axis is, where everything goes round in a circle.

倉廩

Elisabeth Rochat: It's the only time in the presentation of the twelve charges that we have two viscera linked together in order to share the same charge. For all the others we have one viscera for one function. Spleen and Stomach are in charge of storehouses and granaries, *cang lin*. So what is the difference between a storehouse and a granary? It's very difficult. Can we say that the Stomach is more like a storehouse and the Spleen is more like a granary? Or in Chinese the Stomach more *cang* and the Spleen more *lin*? What are the meanings of *cang* and *lin*? It's quite difficult because sometimes the Stomach is called the great

大倉
稟

cang, the great storehouse, and sometimes, for example in Su Wen Chapter 29, we have this kind of sentence, "The twelve viscera, *zang* and *fu*, receive Breaths, *qi*, from the Stomach", and the ideogram which is translated in this context as receive is *lin*. That is very important because in Chinese this ideogram *lin* means not only granaries but also to bring into a place or receive from a place.

Claude Larre: If I may interrupt I would say that the Chinese really have the knack of using the passive or the active form with the same character, so you have to know the doctrine before you make the translation, it's not the translation which gives you the doctrine. Sometimes when they say the active form, to bring, it's good for that context, but the same character will be used for the passive form, and nothing will tell you except your own knowledge. That's the trouble with the Chinese text. But usually, if something has been said in one form, the remainder will be complementary to what has already been said just by way of completion, because you know that everything has to go together.

廩广
府

Elisabeth Rochat: If you look at the ideogram *lin* with the idea of analysis we can see that it is some kind of shelter, a covered place, a barn, or something more important than a barn. If you remember the ideogram for *fu* , you have the same graphic part, it's like a place where you can bring something and place something.

Claude Larre: One could say that it might be a very small shelter with some grain there, or it might be a city itself, which has been made just to keep enough food or materials to distribute to the provinces. The common meaning is that it is a place to store, and then to distribute.

禾回

Elisabeth Rochat: In the character you have the cereals, the stalks of cereal, and a double enclosure with a roof. This is the place where you can bring cereals. But another very common meaning of this ideogram is

6

to make a public distribution of grains, for example during a very hard winter when people are starving the Emperor or the Lord organizes this kind of distribution of the grain. You can see that the important thing is not the Chinese word, or the English word, but all the processes that are implied in that ideogram, i.e. the real use of the granaries as the place which is able to receive and at the same time the place from which the grains are distributed.

 In the case of *cang,* the meaning is of putting together a great quantity of grains in the same place. It's the idea of a meeting, a junction, being together, and that is an appropriate form for the kind of grains we prepare to eat, cooked grains.

The vital thing is to have the idea of this double movement, to receive and then to send to a good place at the right time. Another thing is that this function with a two-fold aspect is linked with the couple or the dual expression, Spleen/Stomach. We can write it Spleen/Stomach in this way in order to call attention to the dialectics of the interplay between Spleen and Stomach, which is really an important aspect of the functioning of the Spleen and Stomach. We will see today and tomorrow that Spleen and Stomach are the best example of the interplay of Heaven and Earth inside the viscera, they are like a turntable - or a revolving platform in the median.

 This is a unique function with a two-fold aspect, and of course, inside that unique function of *cang lin*, storehouse and granaries, we can always think that the Spleen is acting like a *zang,* is actively storing and working on the Essences and their distribution in the depths of the body to all the viscera. And Stomach, acting like a *fu,* is transforming and transporting, and ensuring the passage to the other *fu.*

Spleen and Stomach are working together for the reception, transformation and assimilation of the Essences of alimentation, in order to make the passage into our own vitality and organism. It's another reason for saying that Spleen and Stomach are like a centre, or the go-between, because they are between the exterior (what is exterior to me) and what is mine, my own Essences, or my own organism. They are the intermediary between that which is not me and that which is me. They also act with the help of the other *zang,* like the Essences of the Kidneys, because there is no function or movement which can work in isolation.

The five Tastes and the *jing wei*

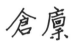

Elisabeth Rochat: What is the effect in the human being of this function of *cang lin,* storing and granaries, and all the processes and movements linked to these two ideograms? The result is that the five Tastes stem from them. I think that you know perfectly well what the five Tastes are, i.e. acid, bitter, sweet, acrid and salty, and that the Taste is not only the taste on the tongue but also all the vitality contained in alimentation which is able to pass into our own vitality through the mechanism of the Essences, or in the state proper to the Spleen and Stomach, *jing wei.* (*jing* for Essences, *wei* for subtle).

What are *jing wei,* subtle Essences? It's the reduction of Essences contained in alimentation, for example from vegetables, cereals or water and their transformation into such a subtle state that these Essences no longer belong to a specific being, to this or that thing that I have eaten, but are able to be composed into the pattern of my own vitality and to become my own Essences. That is *jing wei* - this passage. It's not only in the Spleen and Stomach that we have this kind of passage, but it's above all in the interplay of Spleen and Stomach that we speak of *jing wei.* This, of course, is the same thing as the function of Spleen and Stomach to transform, to assimilate and so on. In the occidental way of speaking it's digestion, assimilation and metabolization: *jing wei* is the classical Chinese expression.

Claude Larre: I have the feeling that we could benefit from coming back to the question of the five Tastes, and clarifying it a little more. When we see vegetables or any sort of food we have the visible sensation of them. Then we prepare them and they are no longer the same as they were, they are closer to assimilation, yet they have the same colour, and we know that they are really leeks or whatever. But as they come closer into our own self, by eating, then the shape, the colour and everything which is really useful to distinguish them is mixed together. But we are not yet at the point of assimilation, and the assimilation when it is done, is done very secretly. The secret is that it is not only the mouth, or the teeth or the Stomach or the organic fluids in the Stomach which are preparing for that, there is something more: there is a function that is so close to oneself, that it is essential. As long as the

五味 *wu wei* (five Tastes) of nature are made in the proper, essential manner it is possible that those external things can become oneself. So, if you are looking at all the process, we understand it is at that point, in that place where nothing can be seen, that the operation of life is taking place.

So coming back to the question of the five Tastes, in the West we call the five Tastes everything that is edible, but the Chinese would call the five Tastes everything which is already assimilated and which might be ranked under those five classes - acid, bitter, sweet, acrid, salty. The

精微 *jing wei* is that particular state of *wu wei* when they are something, but
五味 something which is personal to me. So then for that reason the expression is made up of *jing,* Essences, and *wei,* subtle, because the activity of the Essences cannot be detected by my own means. I am sure by the fact that I am a living person that the activity is very subtle, and that the activity is the activity of life in myself. So the combination of *jing* and *wei* is a sort of abstraction - it's something which is not visible, but which is totally real, which is not a function, but which is some sort of intermediary state of the external five Tastes and the activity I will now be able to display because I have eaten some food.

I am sure that the difficulty in grasping what is said is because it is true! When you think you understand what the point really is, it's certain that you are wrong! Because life is not to be understood. Life is to be an experiment. As long as you are a living person you may see the edible food and you may see the result of your own activity from the fact that you have been nourishing yourself. But in between there is the process of life, and that is what is contained in the meaning of the five Tastes.

Numerology and the number five

Elisabeth Rochat: Five is always whole. It's the entire movement of life in each particular aspect. The doctrine of the ancient Chinese was that we can divide this one unit or unity, this united movement of life, into five main aspects or movements, and on this equal basis we can quite fruitfully observe the entire phenomena of life. That is the foundation and the explanation of what we call the five Phases, or Elements. When we have five, five *zang* or five Tastes, we have the decomposition of a unity into five aspects. For this reason the five Tastes decompose in five different ways the Essences of being. Between Heaven and Earth in this median on Earth, all living beings are in the same pattern so it's for this reason that we have five *zang* and six *fu* and we can breathe the air and eat the fruit of the earth and so on.

Claude Larre: But maybe people will ask since this number five is so good for the *zang* why aren't there five *fu?*

Elisabeth Rochat: It's the same reason as why these five Tastes, with Spleen and Stomach in the hierachy of twelve viscera, in Su Wen Chapter 8, are not in the fifth position, but in the sixth position. In the fifth position we have *tan zhong,* the middle of the chest. *Zhong* is the centre or middle, and *tan* is like an altar from which all the influx of the virtue of the Emperor can radiate to his subjects, his people. This is the altar where the Emperor went each year to call forth the good influence

10

of the Spirits and Heaven, and to be able to make this radiance from the good influx spread to the people. You can see in the fifth position, *tan zhong,* which is also the Sea of Breaths in the middle of the chest, the concentration or the summing up, the gathering of the knot of life in the shape of Breaths. All Breaths are distributed by meridians from the middle of the chest, through the impulse of the Lung and the Earth and the Heart and so on. This is the reason why *tan zhong* is in the fifth position, because these are the Breaths of life, the unity of life, which are used afterwards for rhythmical distribution.

In the sixth position we have Spleen and Stomach with storehouses and granaries. The meaning of six is the maintenance of life. Maintenance is the way of all circulation, alimentation and nutrition in a delineated space. That is quite clearly the function of Spleen and Stomach, to ensure this kind of maintenance. For this reason there are six *fu,* and for this reason Spleen and Stomach are like storehouses and granaries. This vocabulary of storehouses and granaries is very close to the meaning of *fu.*

Spleen and Stomach are in the sixth position in Chapter 8 of Su Wen, and in accord with this the Spleen is very close to the function of the six *fu.* The six *fu* transform and transport in order to present Essences to the viscera, to the body and to the *zang* , so that they can thesaurize (store actively) and release Breaths.

Claude Larre: I feel this is very clear, but in order to make it clearer I would say that my own personal presentation of four, is that the Breaths go Eastward and Westward, Northward and Southward without any organization at all. Then when those expansive Breaths recollect themselves, they come together in order to make a unit, an organized something, five. But when this organized something is done, they go again for expansion, so then it is six. Four and six are understood if we go through number five. Number five is the number of organization. Before five it is four and there is no organization, and after five it is six, and six is just four when four has been organized by passing through five.

11

This is not just a question of numbers. We are **using** numbers. We are using numbers because it is a way for our intellect to understand its own movement. When we are thinking of things we see, or the life we have, we need some sort of presentation of our ideas which are the utmost form of images. Numbers are just images, intellectual images, of our own way of dealing with everything, or the ten thousand beings. When we look at things in themselves, that's objective, and when we are thinking from our own personal self, then we call that our intellectual mode. So numbers are seen in objects or they are seen in our mind. Numbers make our logic, but this logic is not a dream. This logic is encompassing what really exists, and gives a true account of the living beings around ourselves. So the only way for me to understand something is to be intelligent, but to be intelligent I have to make some moves in my mind and those moves are made essentially from numbers. Numbers exist because they are doing something, they are organizing. They exist because they are in myself and I find them again in the external world, so it is impossible to dispense with numbers, we have to accept them and use them. Apart from using these numbers, it is not possible to give an account of the solidity, the firmness, or the validity of the Chinese exposure of life. That's my own personal feeling. Elisabeth was bringing that closer to the subject because she was saying that number six brings Spleen and Stomach towards the other *fu,* so we are more or less leaving the pure activity, and are entering the receptacles, the external vessels through which all life is put.

Elisabeth Rochat: We spoke of six linked with Spleen and Stomach, but the number which is proper to the Spleen is five, of course. We can see that in Su Wen Chapter 4 for example, because in the construction by five through the Spleen is this centre by which the knot, the permutation of Breaths, can take place. Afterwards, it's also the centre from which all *yin* and *yang, zang* and *fu,* six *yin,* and six *yang,* can get maintenance, nutrition, sweet warmth of life and so on. It's always this kind of interplay which is the important point of Chinese spirit, Chinese mind and Chinese physiology.

Gu qi and *jing wei* 穀氣　精微

Question: I would like to have the relationship between *gu qi* and *jing wei* clarified.

Elisabeth Rochat: *Gu qi* are the Breaths of cereals. *Jing wei* is, I think, broader than *gu qi*. *Gu qi* are Breaths coming from alimentation and rising to the Upper Heater in order to compose, with the Breaths coming from respiration, the totality of Breaths of Posterior Heaven circulating in the meridians and so on. The two expressions do not appear at the same time in the history of Chinese medicine.

宗氣
營氣
衛氣
津液

Gu qi doesn't appear in any ancient texts. We speak of *zong qi,* ancestral Breaths, *ying qi,* Breaths with a constructive, nutritional, building function, *wei qi,* defensive Breaths, and so on, but not *gu qi*. *Jing wei* is broader because it's a basis, not only for Breaths, but also for liquids. For example, *jin ye,* body liquids, are based on *jing wei,* and these kind of Essences develop a very great subtlety. *Jing wei,* we saw, is acting between Spleen and Stomach, and sometimes at the level of the Intestines, particularly the Small Intestine, because some kind of assimilation takes place there. But *gu qi* acts at the level of the Sea of Breaths in the middle of the chest, and the circulation and distribution of Breaths through the meridians and the whole network of animation.

The Central Region

The central region is the Earth
The illness is in the Spleen and its *yu* on the spinal column

The yellow aspect of the Earth of the central region
It penetrates and communicates with the Spleen
It opens its orifice at the mouth
It thesaurizes Essences in the Spleen
Thus its disturbance is located at the root of the tongue
Its taste is sweet
Its proper type is earth
Its domestic animal is the ox
Its cereal is millet
Corresponding to the four seasons in the heights it is the planet Saturn
consequently the illness is seen in the flesh
Its note is *gong*
Its number is five
Its odour is aromatic

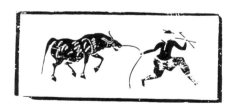

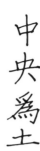

Elisabeth Rochat: Now we can take Chapter 4 of Su Wen, in order to see the first presentation in the Nei Jing of the five *zang* with some of their correspondences, which I prefer to call resonances or harmonics.

First, the Central Region, or *zhong yang*. In English we can say North, West, East, South or Central region, and there is no difference, but in Chinese ideograms there is a difference. For the four directions the Chinese use *fang,* particularly in this text,Chapter 4 and 5 of the Su Wen. It also appears in other books of the same period which are not medical texts but books of rituals, for example, calendars.

Fang means square, which is proper to the Earth. It's proper to the Earth because it's the power, the capacity, and the ability of the Earth to give birth or to make space appear. For this reason a square with four sides is essentially linked with the power of the Earth. In contrast, all the unfolding of time in moments and seasons and so on is concerned with the power of Heaven. So in the spatial sense or meaning, the four directions, *fang,* are like a slice or a portion of space. There is really something defined and delineated with all these spatial qualities. In the North it is cold, hard and frozen, in the South the sun shines , the birds live, and so on. But when you are in the Centre it's impossible to use the same ideogram because it's not exactly the same process. The ideogram *fang* cannot designate the central region, and you find instead *zhong,* the centre (as in *tan zhong)* and another ideogram with the same meaning of a centre, *yang.* In Chinese texts it's impossible to designate

15

方

the five qualities of space by the same ideogram. In Chinese there are only the four *fang* for the directions, never five, but there is a fifth place, a fifth quality of space which is the Central region.

人 口
中
央

Claude Larre: I was looking at Wieger Lesson 60K about *yang,* it says, "A man in the middle of the space". My feeling is that the first character, *zhong,* and the other character, *yang,* are nearly the same character, except that *yang* is more visible than the *zhong. Zhong* is middle and nothing more. *Yang* is the space in the middle which would be occupied by somebody doing something. In some texts we see that the Chinese occupy the central position, and we know that the Chinese consider themselves as the most representative of humanity. So we understand that everything has to be organized from the Centre. The Centre itself can be organized, but somebody has to do the work, and that's the somebody who's in the Centre.

央

Objectively, if you want to command or exert your influence then you have to pick the right place to act from, the Centre. That is where you have to stay and where you have to display your own activity. For that reason, man is represented in the ideogram *yang*. We understand now the big difference Elisabeth was alluding to when she was saying that South, North, East and West are just divisions or portions of space which may have some particular qualities, and the Breaths pertaining to each of those four directions are physically different. But the Centre is distinct because the Centre has all the properties of the four directions, and in harmonizing them it is using them and making everything and everybody servants of itself through its command. So we see that *zhong yang* is not a section of space, it's a place, or even more than a place it's a region - because the Centre is not necessarily a point - the Centre might be a big place, or everything might be the Centre.

中央

Take, for example, international politics. We may say that in the 16th, 17th, or 18th century, France was the Centre of Europe, then England came along and took that position from France. Later on it's no longer Europe that is so important, the United States took the power. So it's true that to be the Centre has nothing to do with geography, but to be the

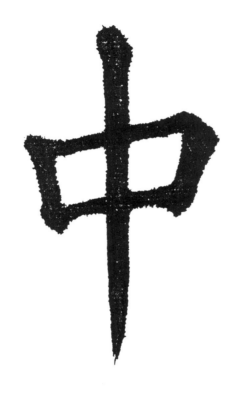

Zhong, the Centre

Centre is to have the power, because you are placed where you can exert that power. The Chinese are not a silly people - they just want to say that being a man you have to occupy the Centre in order to make things move between Heaven and Earth.

土
地

Elisabeth Rochat: In the central region is the Earth, *tu*. You know that the English word 'earth' translates two Chinese words, *tu* and *di*. The difference is that in this case, *tu,* we only have the idea of humus, or soil, with vegetation growing up from it. This ideogram *tu* is used to designate one of the five Elements or Phases, the Element Earth. *Di* has the same idea, but it is also an extension of this power - the idea of the ability to be like a mother. *Di* is Earth as in a couple with Heaven. Heaven is the seed of life and Earth develops this seed and give shape and form to this knot of life and Breaths.

Here in this text it is the first, more simple *tu* which is involved - the Earth as in one of the five Elements, Earth like the soil, a place where men sow and afterwards harvest. If we have a look at old Chinese texts and classical Chinese commentaries when the five Elements or Phases are explained and expounded, the properties of Earth are to receive seeds and afterwards to give harvests. Again we find this two-fold movement of receiving and giving which is exactly the description of the Earth Element in all commentaries.

For example, in commentaries on the Book of History we find the Earth in fifth position. The first position is Water, second is Fire, third for Wood, fourth for Metal, and in the fifth and ultimate position is Earth. The properties of Earth are to receive and give. The Earth can receive all kinds of seeds and give forth all kinds of produce, fruits, cereals and so on, and, of course, all kinds of Tastes, but especially the sweet taste. In the same text just after the enumeration of the Five Elements we have a presentation of the five Tastes. It is the Earth which receives seeds and produces harvests and by that gives comfort in the sweet taste. Sweet is the taste which is able to sum up all the other Tastes.

Claude Larre: If I may add a comment, we usually just have a feeling about taste but we have no description of how they act physiologically speaking. So when Elisabeth says that sweet is at the Centre, and is proper to this condition of Earth, at the same time she is obliged to say why. She said that the effect of sweetness is to recollect, because to recollect is to make things come to the Centre. But it's more a description of how the taste is working than just a description of the feeling you get. This is always a question with Tastes, they are more to be looked at as motions of life than as a feeling we get from eating this or that. There is a distinction between the impression given on the tongue and the true effect of the taste which we get from the edible things which are more or less slowly assimilated into ourselves. This effect is a subtle movement inside our own life-motion. It's always much safer not to consume those five Tastes for the impression we get from them but for their effect - for the differentiation of the movement they have when they are added to our own personal life-motion. Centre, recollect, diffuse, sweet, Earth, all these in themselves are the same. We need a lot of English words, and the Chinese have lots of words too, but essentially, when we go to the actual, the intimate effect, there is one word which is Earth.

Elisabeth Rochat: In the Shu Ji, Book of History, one of the five classics of Chinese literature, the presentation of the five Elements is this order: Water, Fire, Wood, Metal, Earth. The Earth appears through the crossing of the vertical movement from the Water to the Fire with the horizontal movement from the Wood to the Metal. It is the result and the dynamism of the process. A good classical commentary is as follows:

Water and Fire are the solid and liquid foods that the one hundred families look for or seek. Metal and Wood are that by which the one hundred families prosper or can be activated or stimulated. And the Earth is that by which the ten thousand beings have that which is necessary to life, to live.

We can again see this double movement of life, it's the origin of life. We see we have the vital double impulse revealing itself, and taking its vertical position in life with this rising to Heaven in order to attract

Heavenly influx. It's always the same, always with the two-fold aspect. The first movement of life is the springing up, and the second is the activity, the doing of necessary things, between Wood and Metal.

東西
春秋

If we take the directions East and West we have *dong xi,* and *dong xi* is a common expression in Chinese to designate all kinds of things. If we put the seasons Spring and Autumn together we have *chun qiu,* and *chun qiu* in the Chinese is also an old way to designate all kinds of activity. During Winter it's too cold and during Summer it's too hot so these two seasons, Spring and Autumn are periods of activity, for example, making war.

The fifth position is like a Centre and this is Earth. It is that by which the ten thousand beings, or all living beings, have everything they need to live - everything to ensure maintenance and to give life in each moment. In the text it's two Chinese ideograms, one is the ideogram for life, to give birth, to be alive and so on, and the other is the more concrete and material aspect of this maintenance, nourishment and so on. We can see the place of Earth here.

Claude Larre: My own feeling is that there is a very common construction in the sentence. First they state "to be", and to be you need Fire and Water, which is North and South. But to be is to be doing something, acting is really exerting some virtue. This is made from the origin of life, it is made between Spring and Autumn, Wood, and Metal. Spring and Wood are for the vegetation, for the rising movement of plants, and Autumn and Metal are for destruction, the beginning of destruction, war and all that. So, the dual activity is necessarily contained in this rising in the Spring, and receding or falling in Autumn, it couldn't be otherwise. So, after stating what is on the first vertical line, completed by what is on the second horizontal line, at the crossing of those two there is a place to be, and to be active. And this is called Earth. So Earth comes at the end, and at the crossing.

Elisabeth Rochat: You can see from this that Earth is the position which can make both the unity and the diversity. It depends on the point of

20

view. Every living thing returns to the Earth, but, of course, every living being also takes both life and form from that Earth, and for this reason there is a connection with all the varieties of Breath and space and time and so on, in the *zang* and the Tastes.

The Centre, five, Earth, Spleen, the fifth season, which is not exactly a season, all can make the unity of life at this level. And among the seasons, among the spaces, among the Tastes, among everything, universally Earth is also the power through which diversity of shape, of form, of everything can be maintained.

The illness is in the Spleen
and its yu on the spinal column

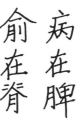

It's quite strange this kind of connection between that which we have just talked about and this illness in the Spleen and the *yu* point. It's because this part of the body, the spinal column, is also a kind of Centre, with an axis where all returns to, and from where all things spread out. You can see that the spinal column is the central part of the body, and it's to the spinal column that all the ribs and muscles and also the viscera are attached.

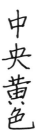

Elisabeth Rochat: When we reach the yellow aspect of the Earth we are at the end of Su Wen Chapter 4, at the place where each of the four directions and the central region are enumerated, with all the proper associations or harmonics of each one. *Huang se* is translated as the yellow aspect of the Earth. There is no ideogram for Earth in the Chinese text, but the colour yellow in Chinese, *huang,* is the special colour of the soil in certain parts of China, especially near the great sinuosity and meandering of the *Huang He* which is the Yellow River. For this reason we sometimes translate not only by "yellow" but with the resonance that this colour has in the Chinese mind. Yellow is the colour of the Earth, the natural colour of the soil.

Claude Larre: It means that yellow is not yellow! Yellow is the colour of the Earth, so it is very clear that it is the Earthy colour which is very akin to what you call yellow.

Elisabeth Rochat: We know that this yellow colour is only the manifested aspect of the fertility of the soil, of the Earth, just as the red colour is not the colour red but the colour of something else, like a fire or something burning. All the time we have to change our own cultural associations to put things into the spirit of the Chinese mind.

Claude Larre: The problem is that the colours that we know are all more or less artificial colours, they are permutations, and they are a product. But what the Chinese are thinking of is the colour of greenery,

22

or the colour of the sky, or the colour of the clouds, or the colour of soil, or the colour of fire, or the colour of water, And if there is no life the colour of the water turns to black. But the black is not what we think of as black, it's more natural - we are in another world where the colour is linked with its efficacy, and to the natural elements. So we have to change our minds in order to recover the knowledge we had formerly.

It penetrates and communicates with the Spleen

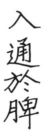

Elisabeth Rochat: Why is this explanation of the yellow colour needed? Because without it we cannot understand the rest of the text.

How can the yellow colour of the Centre or central region penetrate and communicate with the Spleen if we haven't first revised our idea of what yellow is and what the central region is, so that we can understand that the central region is this special function and permutation of Breaths, and also that this yellow aspect is only the visible manifestation of that quality which is the proper quality of the Earth: fertility and stability.

At the same time as the stability there is this capacity for reception, permutation and transformation, and it is this which is the manifestation at the level of the universe of this kind of virtue which can penetrate and communicate with the Spleen, because the Spleen in the human body is exactly the same thing working at the level of the *zang*.

This aspect of the virtue of the universe, of Heaven and Earth and so on, is in resonance, in harmony, and in assonance with all kinds of things or activities in each being which have the same function and quality.

In the human body the five *zang* represent the deeper level, the level of these five qualities of universal life. The Spleen, of course, is in resonance with the yellow aspect of the Earth, the central region. Because the text begins with the Yellow aspect, the first part of this quotation, I think, particularly concerns what is akin with the Essences and qualities of the Earth. Then five lines before the end of the quotation, we have the mention of the four seasons in the heights. I think that the end of the quotation is more akin to the Heavenly aspects of the harmonics and resonance.

It opens its orifice at the mouth

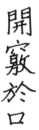

By the mouth all kinds of Tastes penetrate the body, and what are Tastes or cereals or any food but the form or shape of Earthly Breaths?

Claude Larre: All these grains and all that comes forth from the ground under the pressure of Heaven are the materialization of the Earthly Breaths. There is no difference for a Chinese mind between what we call Earthly Breaths and what we see when we look at grains of wheat or rice. We eat them and from that we derive *qi,* which we incorporate into ourselves and use to make our own Breath for our own activity.

The difficulty is not in translation, the difficulty is in having our mind alert and open enough to understand from where the Chinese are drawing all sorts of their statements about *qi.* Why five? Why six? etc. What we have been talking about for two and a half hours was just a preparation for our minds to go deep enough to rejoin the Chinese working on the Breath of the universe and trying to incorporate it through this special mechanism of Spleen and Stomach.

Elisabeth Rochat: We'll see in other chapters, such as Ling Shu Chapter 17, the relationships between the Spleen and its proper orifice, the mouth. But here the focal point is just that we have one of the special qualities of the five aspects of the movement of life, the yellow aspect, penetrating inside the body to reach the deepest level, the *zang*. And the *zang* in harmony with this yellow aspect is the Spleen. After that statement we have the explanation, and the communication between the intimate inside and the exterior in the shape of the orifice.

This opening at the mouth is specially linked with Earth, and the sweet taste of the Earth, and the assimilation, penetration and digestion of the Breaths of Earth in the shape of nutriment and food. Afterwards we come once again to the most intimate aspect of the thesaurization of Essences in the *zang,* in this case the Spleen.

It thesaurizes the Essences in the Spleen

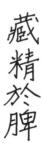

"It thesaurizes" means that it stores actively, because storing is nothing if it is not done actively. Thesaurization is the very stable, quiet and unceasing activity of storing the Essences; that is the function of all the *zang*. All the Essences which are akin with this aspect of life - yellow, central, Earth and so on, are thesaurized by the Spleen. In English or French we must make a choice of saying "by" or "in" the Spleen. In

Chinese we have a single character but the meaning is between the two English words. 'In' the Spleen is too static, 'by' the Spleen is all right - but perhaps the Spleen is not well enough located. Both are good and bad.

Claude Larre: I am sure that since they are talking of the twelve charges, or officials they are talking of some activities, but activities have to have a place. It's a question of Heaven and Earth. The activity is more related to the Heavenly flux, but the Heavenly flux has to fall somewhere in order to be effective, So when Elisabeth was talking about this question of grammar or translation, should we say 'by' or 'and' or 'in' or 'inside', it's true that the only important thing is the active connection between the Essences and the Spleen, and there is no active connection if there is no place for that. But place itself is not just a place, place is the *yin* aspect of this *yang* activity. Or maybe the reverse? It is impossible to tell where the knot of life is made. We may make some sort of exploration of what happens, but there is never a point when we can say it is this and truly not that. We are exploring something which is written and we are sent back to our own experience. If we have been treating people using Stomach and Spleen according to what we have been taught and what they are, we know more than people who have only been reading the text. But the text itself sends you back to the effect of life which you know yourself, and by the treatment you have been giving people. There lies the explanation. It's always best to be sent back to life.

藏
神魂魄
意 志

Elisabeth Rochat: The *zang* is an active function and at the same time a dwelling place for Essences. This is said in the text, but behind the Essences we have Spirits or higher entities ie. *shen, hun* and *po* or *yi* and *zhi.* In the case of the Spleen it is *yi,* but we'll see that later in other chapters of the Su Wen and Ling Shu.

26

Thus its disturbance is located
at the root of the tongue

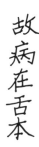

Because of the connection between Spleen and the root of the tongue, it is the place where certain diseases connected with trouble in the thesaurization of the Essences by the Spleen can appear. The root of the tongue is just at the level where the external manifestation of the power of the internal thesaurization of the Essences by the Spleen takes place. This is the meaning of the sentence. It does not mean all diseases caused by the Spleen are at the root of the tongue. Of course, in the case of diseases of the Spleen we can also have some disturbance of taste.

Its taste is sweet

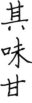

If we look at the etymological interpretation of sweet in Wieger lesson 73B, we can see that the ideogram for sweet is very simple - it is just a hand and a mouth. So the etymological explanation of sweet is any kind of thing which can be held in the mouth and gives satisfaction.

Sweet is one of the five Tastes and its place is in the Centre. It is the summing up of all kinds of taste which are able to give satisfaction

27

because they are a good balance or in good harmonization, without poisons for the body. Sometimes poisons have a very good taste, but perhaps if you are really 'authentic' or if you have a good feeling of what you are, you can feel the poison. I personally can not!

Its proper type is Earth

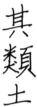

Five is Earth, *tu*. The ideogram is not the ideogram of the Element or agent as in the five Phases or Elements. In this case, Earth is a type of species *lei,* like man belongs to the human species. It's the species of mouth, Spleen, of Essences stored in the Spleen, of sweet, and so on. Of all these aspects Earth is a great type, a fundamental pattern of distribution of all things over the Earth within five categories.

Its domestic animal is the ox

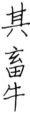

This fits in with all the things we have said - that the ox is working the Earth all the time, and oxen have a colour which is similar to the yellow aspect of the Earth. For the Chinese mind the ox is not red or green, it's yellow. Also the association is a very old Chinese idea. I'll read a quotation from the Records of History, which is a great Chinese book written one hundred years BC:

The ox is in fact the one who labours and works, who plants and sows in order to make things exist. He labours, plants and sows the ten thousand kinds of creatures in order to make things exist.

We have the same explanation of the qualities of Earth in other texts and we can see in the Chinese mind how these kinds of harmonics have exactly the same real active qualities, and we can use a similar vocabulary. The ox isn't the one who plants and sows, but he's the one who works in order that this can take place. But the Chinese text says that the ox plants and sows. This is because the ox works in the same way that the Earth works, or the Spleen and so on; and the ox is like the slave girl, very docile, very stable and even tempered. It's not like a race horse, and it's not like a mole sleeping under the Earth, it's between the two. This good tempered aspect is also a quality of Earth and Spleen and Stomach and so on, Spleen and Stomach are not too hot and not too cold, not too dry and not too humid.

Its cereal is millet

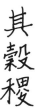

Its cereal is millet, *ji,* panicled and non-glutinous. One thing that is important is that this name *ji* is also the name of the Chinese god of agriculture Hou ji, Prince Millet. He's the deity of the harvest, of cereals and agriculture, and there is a famous poem about him and his marvellous birth in the Book of Odes, which has a good English translation by Arthur Waley. And, of course, this millet is yellow!

29

I think we can read the rest of the quotation from Su Wen Chapter 4 quite quickly because the main points are also found in the next chapter.

Corresponding to the four seasons in the heights it is the planet Saturn

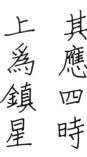

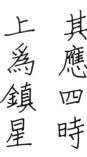

Its virtue in Heaven is seen in the influence of Heaven on time and movement, moment and season. But how can Heaven manifest its proper essences in the shape of five planets? One way is the form of this manifested aspect such as the colour of each of the planets: Mars is rather red, Venus rather shiny, and so on. It is the planet Saturn that manifests the kind of virtue akin to the Spleen and Stomach. An ideogram for planet could be *xing,* which is the same ideogram which on Earth designates the *wu xing,* or five Phases. It has exactly the same qualities. In order to explain this strange, bizarre sentence to an occidental mind, with this planet corresponding to the four seasons in the heights, we need to see that it is the expression of the vitality of Heaven expressed in five different qualities, just as we can see *yin* and *yang* in Heaven in the shape of the sun and moon. So in Heaven there is also a possibility of dividing the unity into five aspects, five qualities of Breaths, or virtues, and you can see therefore that there are five planets. On the other hand, if the Earthly power organizes space, the Heavenly power creates time.

***Consequently the illness
is seen in the flesh***

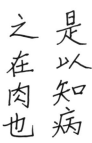

Flesh gives the shape of the body, and it is the power of the Earth that can give form to ideas and shape to the disease which is proper to the body. Flesh is not just this mass-giving shape, but also a place where all kinds of circulation can take place. Flesh is penetrated by ravines and valleys and all kinds of pathways, and this is the kind of circulation by which we find the shape again. The cohesion of man is given more by the void allowing circulation and relationships rather than by compact density.

Its note is the note gong

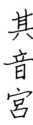

The note *gong* is used as a basis for all the other notes. It is the first note of the pentatonic scale, and the first note is a basic note.

Its number is five

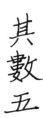

We saw this quality of five to be the crossing of flux coming from the four directions into a Centre between Heaven and Earth, or *yin* and *yang*. This is five, and this is the Spleen acting like a revolving platform. We shall see later this function of the Spleen and Stomach in the raising and lowering, ascending and descending movement of all things, and the distribution of Breaths and separating of clear and unclear and so on.

Its odour is aromatic

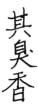

Aromatic, *xiang,* is perhaps like sweet in being an harmonious composition of Breaths. It is one of the five kinds of dividing odours - an odour which gives satisfaction, but a satisfaction that comes from this feeling of something balanced and well harmonized with a good composition, compenetration and permutation of Breaths. It is the same in the odours as in Tastes.

Claude Larre: It seems that sweet and aromatic are the same thing, but diffusing in different ways. When you are in the country in August and

32

everything is smelling in an aromatic way it is because the atmosphere is full of the odours of the crops or the plants under the sun, but if you were not there to experience that, the taste would still be there inside each grain or each plant. So, for myself, I feel that they first say something about the taste and then they go forward from the innermost to the most outward effect which is the odour.

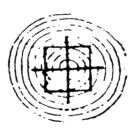

Summary

脾 胃

Claude Larre: Yesterday we started with drawings and explanations of the two ideograms *pi* and *wei,* trying to see them in their interplay and marking how *pi* and *wei* join together in order to make some sort of vital Centre. We have also been observing that life, being a compenetration of influxes, is always at the meeting point, in the median, where Heaven and Earth make connection. And since life is a gift, life has to be received, and its central place, seen in an individual, is in the Spleen and Stomach. In every living being (and by living being we are not talking only of animals, it's also true of plants and it's true of the universe itself) there must always be the same analogical structure repeating itself everywhere. So be it in me, in you, in human kind, in the animal kingdom, or in the universe, there is always a meeting point, or a place where this secret meeting of life takes place, and there is no room for intellectual explanation except by coming back to the division of the roles of Heaven and Earth. But actually what exists, what is making us, *hic et nunc,* is not to be seen and not to be described. We are just observing the contours of it, and by seeing how somebody in good health is, we try to understand how this silent process works. At the same time if something goes wrong, then we start observing something and hearing some different sounds. So it is always easier to describe something which is going astray than to describe the normal condition of life.

脾藏
胃府

As for the relation of *pi* being a *zang,* and *wei* being a *fu* we may use different dialectics. The prime dialectic, I don't say the easiest, but the most obvious, is *yin yang.* Then we may consider using another set of dialectical principles, the five Elements or Phases, which are essentially the same as *yin yang,* but *yin yang* seen as the beating of life, the rising of the *yang,* the sliding of the *yang* and the coming up of the *yin.* We may see all that as life beating between *yin* and *yang.* Or we may see how a particular being tries to organize itself, and then this *yin yang* system does not give enough light for our understanding. We have to pass on to a more elaborate vision, which is to enter the question of how

34

脾 胃

the so-called five Elements or five Phases are situated one with the other. In this particular case, if we are describing the interplay between *pi* and *wei* we have to know which Element we would choose as the reference Element for the interplay of *pi* and *wei*. Obviously it's the fifth Element, but why do we say the fifth and not the first, second or third? Is there an order or not?

中央

膻中
脾胃

When we read Chapter 4 and Chapter 5 of Su Wen, we see that *zhong yang,* the central region, is in the third place, and that in this set of five propositions it occupies the Centre. But when we look at Chapter 8 of the Su Wen we see that Spleen and Stomach come at the end of the first series: Heart, Lung, Liver, Gall Bladder, *tan zhong,* and *pi wei.* So there is no difference, it's just the presentation which is not the same. In any case our main teaching is that we are trying to explain how there is a Centre for this Breath which is making our own life, which can be distinguished from the life of the universe but at the same time shouldn't be. The highest mystery in our own personal life is that we feel so strongly that we are in opposition to, or distinct from everything which is not our own self, and at the same time we are called back to the nature of our life which is just an expression of the universe. But there is no contradiction in that because every contradiction is just a part of life's movement and is not so easily solved by our mind's understanding of things.

Now, to say something a little more about this question of the Centre. Yesterday I was saying that the Heart might be taken as a Centre because everything is ruled by the Heart. But the Heart is more than a Centre, it is at the same time the sovereign of life. In another context, the Centre is occupied by something which is not the Heart, but which maintains life through the absorption of whatever might be used for that. I need some device to absorb the *qi* of the universe and to make my own *qi* from that *qi* , and that device is the combination of *pi* and *wei,* Spleen and Stomach.

氣
脾胃

肝 膽

If I put two Chinese characters together making a dual expression, I may see them in opposition, in likeness or in compenetration. In Zhuang Zi Chapter 2 *gan dan,* Liver and Gall Bladder are shown to be so close that they almost seem the same, but they are also so different, that they could be said to be as different as Beijing and Hong Kong. Zhuang Zi Chapter 2 was written in the fourth century BC, so it seems that the concept of being close and being opposed, being one unit, is really something that the Chinese mind had at an early time, before the Su Wen or any medical text was known to be written. So, three, or four or five centuries before Christ, the Chinese were able to see, and tell us clearly and without error or clumsiness, how what are opposite may also compenetrate and become the living factor of life.

脾胃

氣

What, then, is really the function of *pi wei,* Spleen and Stomach? It's that when life has been given, life has to be fed and renewed, and we need some nutritional elements. But to take them from the universe we need some selector, or selective device, related to our own Essences, some sort of capacity in ourselves to choose what is convenient and neccessary and to discard what is not. One may say that the Small Intestines, or even the Large Intestines are there for that. In a way they are, but in a very auxiliary way. The highest power to make the selection from the *qi* of the universe and to present it to oneself is in the charge of the Spleen, with the association of all the others, because nothing works independently. The ordinary presentation of life is the association of the *zang* with the *fu,* so what sort of *fu* has to be in association with the Spleen in order to make this selection of what is really similar to and necessary for our own Essences? It is the Stomach, and it will be seen now through the teaching of Elisabeth, how that is understood, not in the generalities of yesterday, but in the practicalities of the text which give the description of the subtle physiology, and how the meridians are working together. And we will see how when something goes wrong we need to intervene to try to restore some kind of equilibrium in order that this selection process will go on - to prevent the Stomach reflecting its own disorder in the highest activities of man's life.

Most of us have friends who have died from cancer, and we know how they can have pain in the stomach and how they are disturbed in their mind. So we know the connection between the disorder in the Spleen and Stomach and the disorder in the governing or meditative power which is a Centre for the mind. So if the Stomach and Spleen are not doing what they are supposed to do there will be the same disorder on a higher level as there is on a more physical and physiological level. There will be suffering and premature death, and at the same time there will have been a sort of loss of taste for life, something will go astray because the unity of life is lost.

So, we are just here to see how the Chinese have seen life and how they've been able, in this complexity of life, to make the distinction between so many working places or so many agents, and to ascribe to each of them specific behaviour, to observe all those exchanges of energy and try to give an explanation for all disorders.

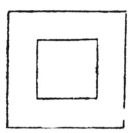

SU WEN CHAPTER 5

The central region produces Dampness....

The central region produces dampness
Dampness produces Earth
Earth produces the sweet
Sweet produces the Spleen
Spleen produces the flesh
Flesh produces the Lung
The Spleen is master of the mouth

That which in Heaven makes dampness
On Earth makes the earth
In the body makes the flesh
In thesaurization makes the Spleen
In the coloured aspects makes yellow
In the notes makes the note *gong*
In the noises makes singing
In movements reacting to change makes eructations
In the orifices makes the mouth
In the Tastes makes the sweet
In the instances of will makes meditative thought

Meditative thought injures the Spleen
That which victoriously balances out meditative thought is anger
Dampness injures the flesh
That which victoriously balances out dampness is wind
Sweet injures the flesh
That which victoriously balances out sweet is acid

Elisabeth Rochat: We continue with Chapter 5 of the Su Wen which shows another way of giving the relationships of the Earth Element with the Spleen and other functions in the body. We saw in Chapter 4 of the Su Wen the central region and the yellow aspect of the Earth in connection with the Spleen and its Essences, and with all the things in the universe which have the same quality of Breath, such as domestic animals, cereals and so on. Now in Su Wen Chapter 5 we look more precisely at the human body.

The central region produces dampness

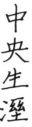

What is the meaning of that, and how can the central region produce dampness? It must be because the central region, like the Earth Element, has the quality of being able to receive - to receive good irrigation in watering, good seeds and richness. And at the same time it has the ability to give forth something, to give birth, to produce cereals and so on and to give other things food, cereals or irrigation. In the Chinese tradition the explanation of the central region producing dampness is that the central region has the ability to water the four directions, the four sides of space. It's like a reservoir. In the same manner the end of the Summer is that special period when the warmth brings up the humid Breaths of the Earth for evaporation. It's the idea of the Earth penetrated with dampness and humidity and worked on by the warmth, so that at the end of the Summer you arrive at this stage of damp Breaths which evaporate, and the warm vapours rising from the Earth give form and shape to clouds, and that makes rain and dew. As a result we have the fertility of Earth, and cereals can be produced. So this humidity of Earth, or of the central region is the ability to be very fertile.

Dampness produces Earth

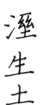

Perhaps this is because Earth, humus, soil, dampness or central region are a place or a function where all kinds of things can simmer together in order to release good Breaths for the maintenance of *yin* and *yang, zang* and *fu,* all the meridians and so on. It is also because Earth, or humus, or soil, mixed with dampness, is the best way to give form to something - like pottery. With the Earth, which has been worked on by dampness, there's the idea that something could be modelled or formed into something. The idea of fertility is this idea of taking shape and form together, and we saw that the great function of the Earth Element is to give form by transformation. So it's exactly the same for the Spleen inside the body.

Earth produces the sweet

We saw previously the relationship between Earth and sweet: that Earth produces sweet in that the Earth producing cereals, and all kinds of food, produces at the same time the well-harmonized composition of these Breaths of food. That is the basic meaning of what is sweet. It's by the function of Earth simmering things together that we have sweet. Sweet, as a taste, is here at the highest level, it's like a basic structure which appears between Heaven and Earth (Earth with the meaning of *di).* For this reason, "Sweet produces the Spleen"

40

Sweet produces the Spleen

甘
生
脾

The pattern of sweet can also be the inner pattern for this function which in the body is called the Spleen. And of course, in a healthy body, the food which contains Essences with sweet qualities can maintain and renew the function of the Spleen.

Spleen produces the flesh

脾
生
肉

The meaning of this sentence is that this activity which we awkwardly call Spleen, and which is basically a function, expresses itself through all the levels of the structure of the body or the person, through thought and through physical structures and in bodily structures is just flesh. Flesh gives form to the body, and flesh is the place for the circulation of all Breaths and all nutrition, and this circulation reaches to the extremity of the four limbs. We have flesh in the general form of the body but within the flesh we can also see large and small valleys. This is very interesting because the ideogram for valley, *gu,* is an homophone with the ideogram for cereals, *gu,* and sometimes in modern Chinese the ideogram for valley is used as the abbreviated form for the ideogram for cereals. Breaths of cereals and Breaths of a valley are not exactly the same, of course, but there is a natural link between them both. If cereals, by the activity of the Stomach and Spleen, can give form to the body through the flesh, flesh itself has specific forms, for example the form of each muscle. There are muscular valleys and all the inner, smaller valleys which penetrate into the mass of the flesh and enable all kinds of circulation - of Blood and *qi* and so on.

I think this is another example of the two-fold aspect of activity and stability of the Earth: to have form and transformation at the same time, because it's impossible to have life or form without transformation. Of course you know that if our Breaths and the activity of the Spleen are in a well-balanced state, our flesh will be in a good state. All the activity of the Spleen in transporting Breaths, liquids and nutritional Elements through the body means that flesh should be in good form.

Flesh produces the Lung

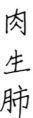

Next we have this quite bizarre sentence "Flesh produces the Lung". We have to understand how Spleen or Earth or all these aspects of the movement of life, can produce Lung or Metal. We can see how the power and strength of Earth, through the Spleen, can make the Essences and Breaths of the Middle Heater rise up into the Upper Heater and give the Lung the opportunity to distribute Breaths rhythmically through all the body. So, of course, the Lung needs these Essences and Breaths of food to fulfil its task. There is a very common Chinese expression: "Spleen is the source for the production of Breaths and Lung is the pivot for the Breaths".

The relationship between Lung and Spleen is very close, of course, because they are both *tai yin*. We see in Su Wen Chapter 11 that the explanation of the importance of the pulse on the meridian of *tai yin* of the hand is also linked to the function of the Spleen, the *tai yin* of the foot. But in Chapter 5 we have "Flesh produces the Lung", and it's quite strange. The meaning is that one Element, and one *zang* can produce, give birth and life to another *zang* or Element through its own activity and its own production. Flesh is a product of Spleen when the resonances of Spleen are manifested, because we can see and touch the flesh - but it is very difficult to be in touch with the Spleen, because the Spleen is not exactly a visible mass. Yet because the function of the Spleen can manifest its virtue in the flesh of the body we can have a real effect which produces the other Element or *zang,* and helps this other Element or *zang* to fulfil its task.

In the presentation of Su Wen Chapter 5 this is absolutely systematic, in the case of Liver, and the East and so on, we have the Liver producing muscle and muscle producing the Heart. In the case of the South, Heart produces Blood, and Blood produces Spleen. This sentence "Blood produces Spleen" can be interpreted as the Blood of the Heart bringing to the Spleen all that it needs to be well nourished, and the spiritual orientation which is necessary for the power of the Earth and the Spleen. Also, the Heart which is master of the movement of circulation and animation of the Blood inside the body brings the Spleen the possibility of having this movement of distribution for liquids and nourishing Breaths etc.. Perhaps the relationship between the movement of the Spleen and the movement of the Lung takes place thanks to the flesh, because if we see the flesh as being overrun with valleys and ravines, what are valleys and ravines but channelways for the circulation of Breaths which are distributed from the Lung and the centre of the chest?

生

Claude Larre: One of the difficulties of explaining this section of Chapter 5 is that the Chinese character *sheng* is used six times to make a connection between two aspects. The first is that the central region gives birth to, produces, makes appear, or makes come forth, humidity. And life is produced through humidity, but humidity itself has to be somewhere. Humidity might be in the sky, but the humidity for making life come forth has to be the equivalent of Earth. First humidity, then Earth, for the producing of life. If we want to see grass we need humidity and we need humus. Life is produced as life in itself by the fact that there is no difference between the central region and humidity. When we say *sheng* we must understand the producing of life starts, as far as the central region is concerned, from humus, and then we can progress to another connection between central region, humidity and Earth. Then we come to what Earth is for ourselves, and the Earth for oneself is the Spleen. Each time we move from one stage of life to the next we are coming nearer to ourselves, because man is the Centre of the operation of Heaven and Earth, and the organizational factors of life are the *zang*. Here the *zang* chosen is the Spleen.

A more internal view of the same thing is that *qi* has to be somewhere, and the *qi* which makes life more and more powerful is in the valleys and ravines inside the flesh. The flesh is much more full of empty spaces than solid places. The solid places are just there to relieve the interval spaces for the *qi*. As we used to say in molecular or atomic work, there's much more void in this table than it seems there is, and even in titanium and uranium, which are the heaviest metals, there is enough void to draw the energy which is there. So there is a connection between void and energy, so much so that to speak of the movement of life we have to speak of flesh, and speaking of flesh we are speaking of those places where energy is resting and is ready to be used. That was the reason why Elisabeth was talking so much about flesh, not visible flesh, but flesh for the emptiness, which is a requisite for life.

And all this is connected with *sheng,* because in those empty places full of Breaths there is production - production of the organ through which the animated Breaths are regulated, the Lung. The Lung is the chancellor of life, the highest administrator of life, the Prime Minister over all the other ministers, because the only point of being a living being is to manage well the Breaths that we have, both the Breaths we first received and the Breaths we draw from outside to build and replace what has been exhausted by our own activity. When we come to the seventh sentence of this section of Su Wen Chapter 5, it no longer uses

生
脾

the *sheng* character but another one, *zhu.* So six characters make the relationship between two sets of characters using *sheng:* the central region and humidity, humidity and the Earth, Earth and sweet, sweet and *pi, pi* and flesh, flesh and Lung. So how do we feel about the fact that there are six relationships here?

Elisabeth Rochat: Two for Heaven, two for Earth and two for Man.

Claude Larre: Yes, most probably there are six because Heaven, Earth and Man are in relation, so 3 x 2 is 6. That's obvious, but it has to be verified, and you have to see if it gives something. We are not supposed to make mechanical explorations of the text, but we are using mechanical exploration of the text to see if we understand more or less. If we understand more then we can say it is intended to show this and that, and if it doesn't tell us anything then we drop it.

生

All this is to make you understand that when using this *sheng* character, to produce or give birth, we are obliged, by means of our own imaginary power, to change the English translation because if we just say to produce or give birth, the connection between Lung and flesh is not seen. It's easier to say that the Earth is producing something than to say that the flesh is producing the Lung.

生

Elisabeth Rochat: Sheng is not only to produce and give birth but also to maintain life, or life itself, and the fact of being alive.

Claude Larre: The fact is that life itself wants to go on, so between 'to live' and 'to maintain' there is no difference where life is concerned.

45

Spleen is master of the mouth

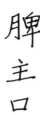

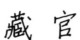

Elisabeth Rochat: We saw that previously. But this is not a relationship of producing or giving birth, it is a relationship of mastering because the mouth is like a servant of an overlord, and the overlord is the Spleen. The lord and king is the *zang* and the orifice is like an official, *guan*.

That which in Heaven makes dampness on Earth makes the Earth

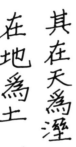

What is 'that'? 'That' is the mystery of life, the mysterious transformation of the influence of the Spirits of Heaven into what happens on Earth and to all the ten thousand living beings. This 'that' is the mysterious heart of life which we can never express or explain; but we can see five rays of light springing out of this unlabelled mystery of life. If we look at one of these rays we see the central region, dampness, soil, flesh, Spleen and so on, with a very organic link between them. In the same way when you play a musical note on certain instruments you can hear all the harmonics of that note. It is the same. Look at these rays of light, and like harmonics I can see all that we call correspondences. They are organic, vital, living - exactly like this because they are not correspondences but the same movement of life.

46

土 地

So we know that that which in Heaven makes dampness, which is one of the six aspects of the unique Breath of Heaven, on Earth, *di,* makes the Earth, *tu,* one of the Five Elements.

...in the body makes flesh...

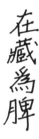

...the form of the body and the place for circulation of Breaths and Blood and so on.

...in thesaurization makes the Spleen...

...the great thesaurizer of permutations of all kinds of Breaths, of transformation, transportation and nourishment.

...in the coloured aspects makes yellow

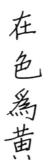

...the colour that you see in millet, and that you can see if you look at loess, the Yellow River and so on.

...in the notes makes the note gong

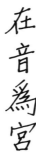

This is the first note of the pentatonic scale, and the basis for the elaboration of the other notes.

在聲爲歌

音 聲

聲

What is the difference between notes, *yin,* and noises, *sheng* ? Notes are a celestial vibration. The five notes are a typical example of this division by five, and the five notes are very close to the numbers. A complex and subtle play of numbers establishes each of the five notes in its own length of vibration. [See Granet. La Pensee Chinoise]. Numbers are invisible and untouchable, but they are real because through numbers and numerology you can understand the way in which Heaven and Earth build life, and the inner pattern of life. And notes are something like this in the field of vibration. Notes are the pattern that we can't hear, but through which we can understand the building of all sound. These five notes allow all kinds of music, through sounds that you can hear. Noise, *sheng,* is quite difficult to express in French or English, but it's the sound that you hear when the vibration is passing through a tube, like a musical pipe. In this case the pipe, or the musical instrument is not a piano or a harpsichord or bagpipes, it's our own body.

When sound which is in harmony with the first note, with Earth, Spleen and so on, passes through our body like a pipe, it is singing. Why singing? Because when all is well harmonized, when we are full of satisfaction, as with sweet and aromatic, we are happy, and the natural expression of that is singing. You know that Spleen is linked with thought or thinking, and if you are thinking you are thinking of something, and this is very near to having the desire for something. If you can realize your desire you are happy, and you sing. It's also that there's good connection between Spirit and Essences through the good harmonization of all thinking and willing and Breaths and Essences which come from all directions and are well harmonized in the Centre. When that happens, you simply sing.

...in movements reacting to change
makes eructations

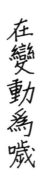

Up until now it has all been a description of the normal way of things, but now we have a description of a reaction to a bad change, an inversion of the normal situation. If the aggravation affects the aspect of life near the Spleen, then as a result we have this kind of response, eructations, which are a counter-current movement of the Stomach, and the too quick and violent rising up of the Spleen. This is pathological, although usually it's not very serious. Sometimes you can simply have this kind of eructation because you ate too quickly, or too much. In fact it's very polite in China to have a little eructation after a good dinner. If you just say, "It was such a delicious dinner, my dear," that's not enough, you have to manifest that it is really true by this inner movement of your Spleen.

...in the orifices makes the mouth
...in the Tastes makes sweet

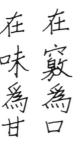

We won't remain longer on this issue.

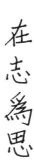

志

五志

Zhi is linked with the Kidneys, but here we have instances of will for each of the five *zang*. If *zhi,* the will, is the vital tension of life inside the deepest foundation of life, Kidneys, then we can also see this tension of life at the level of each *zang*. In this case we speak of the five wills, *wu zhi,* and the meaning is that which is, at the mental or emotional level, the expression of the vital tension of each *zang*. And for the Spleen we have these meditative thoughts. For the Liver we have anger, which is not exactly the kind of anger which we see as an expression of a certain kind of violence, it is more like a vital impulse. For the Heart it is elation, not joy but elation, which can be very, very good allowing the circulation of Blood and Breaths throughout all the network of animation. But if this elation is too strong it can be very dangerous and can release the vital sources, the Essences, Breaths and Spirits. But in the case of the Spleen we have meditative thought.

心

囟

意

We saw this kind of thought when we studied Ling Shu Chapter 8. The ideogram is made up of heart, and in the upper part the primitive representation of the brain. The classical explication of this ideogram is that if the Spirits of the Heart are in good communication with the brain you can have thought. This belongs to the Spleen, of course, because the Spleen takes care of the maintenance and renewal of Essences, and the Essences permit the Spirits to express themselves. If you remember Ling Shu Chapter 8, the purpose, *yi,* is the first process which appears when the Heart is acting. When we have a Centre to take charge of all beings, the first thing the Heart can do is apply itself, and this application of the Heart to what is presented is *yi. Yi* is a superior activity of the Spleen, of the Earth, of the Centre of the body and so on.

The text of Ling Shu Chapter 8 continues:

When the will that remains changes at the same time, that is thought.

The meaning is that you can have attention and will, like the vital impulse and attention to something or somebody, but that is not thought. Thought appears when through that attention and with this will, you are able to look at other possibilities and to look at the very best way to realize something. It's not that the will changes like a weather vane, but it's like a good consideration of the diverse aspects of the situation, while you remain very firmly on the way to something. That is thought.

Claude Larre: It's more or less circling the issue that you want to do something about. First you have this something which is like a point. But that something has to be enriched by consideration while you are still with your own will, which is fixed on that object. But you are able to set your mind free and keep your will. So at the same time there is this constant will and there is a free circulation of the Breaths within around your intention, so to speak. This complex situation is thinking thought.

Elisabeth Rochat: You can see that both stability and transformation are necessary for thinking - which is just a refinement of the fundamental notions or processes linked with the Earth, the Spleen and so on. If you remember the text of Ling Shu Chapter 8, after the becoming of thoughts there is the ability for them to spread out far and wide very powerfully. Afterwards, as a result, you have *lu,* reflection, meditation, planning and projection. We can find in this spreading out far and powerfully the expression of what we, rather later, call the *yang* of the Spleen, the ability to distribute and transport and so on. You can understand now why, when in pathological terms we say the *yang* of the Spleen is not enough, thought and reflection are disturbed and weak. It's exactly the contrary of being able to go far and powerfully. If the *yin*

of the Spleen Essences are not enough then thinking is poor and you lose your memory because there is no longer the presentation of something to the Spirit of the Heart, and the Spleen is no longer able to give or to maintain forms in thinking, such as ideas and memories.

Meditative thought injures the Spleen

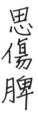

At the end of Su Wen Chapter 5 you have the pathological aspect of these meditative thoughts. When meditative thought is unable to go far and powerfully the thought turns around, and in this case meditative thought injures the Spleen. There is no distribution, there is no giving of form, just churning something over and over. Meditative thought turns into worries and concerns.

That which victoriously balances out meditative thought is anger

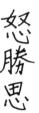

In the *ke* cycle you have this, but what is the meaning of the *ke* cycle? It's that anger is the expression of the vital impulse which goes far and powerfully, because it's exactly the meaning of Liver, Wood, East, Spring and so on. This is exactly the function of Liver in the organism, and exactly the definition of anger in the emotions. For this reason anger can give good balance to meditative thought which lacks this movement and ability to go far and powerfully. You can see it in terms of movement and quality of Breaths.

Claude Larre: As for anger, you know 'anger' is one of the English words used for translating the character *nu,* but it would be wise to forget so-called anger, and think of any sort of violent movement with this vital force or strength. Conventionally we call it anger, but behind the English word we must understand that it is the vital strength acting on this meditative mood which counterbalances it and may restore the force you need to think things over and achieve your aim.

Elisabeth Rochat: The meaning of this sentence is not that if someone is depressed because of their Spleen you have to make them angry in order to cure them!

Claude Larre: But it is true that it works!

Elisabeth Rochat: True sometimes! But its aim is to restore in the person this aspect of the movement of life at the level of the emotions, because it's at the level of the emotions that the person is disturbed.

54

Dampness injures the flesh

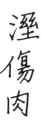

We have exactly the same schema with dampness and wind. Dampness injures the flesh because dampness provokes a kind of loosening in the flesh, a flaccidity, and there is no longer any transformation, movement and circulation.

That which victoriously balances out dampness is wind.

Wind balances out this kind of over abundant dampness because wind can dry, and it can establish circulation again so there's no more blockage. The wind can sweep things aside. These are the qualities of wind we find in the Chinese text.

Question: What is the character for 'victoriously balances'?

Elisabeth Rochat: Sheng. Sheng is to dominate. This is the ideogram

55

刳
勝 生

which is often used in the Nei Jing instead of *ke,* as in the *ke* cycle. *Ke* appears very few times in the Nei Jing, usually you have this ideogram *sheng*. *Sheng* is a homophone of the other *sheng,* to give birth, to produce and so on - so we have two cycles, *sheng* and *sheng*. To dominate is a very common and useful ideogram. It's used for seasons, for Elements, for all things which dominate each other, in the manner of the so called *ke* cycle. This ideogram *ke* is a little bit stronger and a little more aggressive than *sheng*.

Claude Larre: We must mention that the two *sheng* characters have a different tone, and the Chinese would not consider this to be a homophone if the tone is not the same. *Sheng* is a victory and a victory has something calm about it because the work is done, so victory is equivalent to peace. But to repress or to conquer is *ke* , so there is a difference in the feeling the Chinese may have when they are talking of *ke* and when they are talking of *sheng*. One is more aggressive and repressive, and the other is just the fact that now things come back to order through the intervention of something very powerful which counterbalances what was going astray.

Elisabeth Rochat: Perhaps the explanation is very simple. In the Nei Jing Chapter 5 the focus point is essentially on the exposition of the deep and intimate inner mechanism of normal life, and the pathological aspect is just the disturbance and imbalance of this normal life. In the commentaries and other medical books the focus is on the diversity of pathological aspects and their treatment, and in this case *ke* is a good word because the person is ill and there is a *ke* effect, not only a *sheng* effect, which is the succession and equilibrium of all things, sometimes with disturbance, of course. So this is the ideogram which is translated 'victoriously balances out'.

Sweet injures the flesh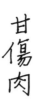

According to the Nei Jing too much sweet has an effect of loosening the flesh and the result of loosening is bad circulation because there is no impulse and no tension for circulation.

That which victoriously balances out sweet is acid

For this reason what victoriously balances out sweet is acid, because the property of acid is to draw together or shrink, it has an astringent quality.

Question: You said that dampness injures the flesh and gives a flaccidity, now the sweet injures the flesh and loosens it, so could you explain what the difference is?

 Elisabeth Rochat: Dampness and sweet are exactly the same at the level of the Breaths of Heaven or the Tastes of the Earth, *qi* and Essences and so on, so their effects must be the same according to the level of reality and the property of *qi*, Breaths of Heaven and Tastes. The result is something very similar because we are in exactly the same harmonic. Sometimes the same vocabulary can be employed by the Chinese as we saw with the Earth and the ox, for example.

57

Claude Larre: I will take ten minutes to review all this and try to see how this description in Su Wen Chapter 5 is coherent. First, I don't feel they are talking of Heaven for Heaven's sake, or Earth for Earth's sake, it seems to me that it is the same wording and the same representation as we saw when they say in Ling Shu Chapter 8:

Heaven in me is virtue

In Ling Shu Chapter 8 are they talking of Heaven or me? They are talking of me, but they say that the presence of Heaven constitutes the initiative for having self, and it is the virtue of Heaven which makes the appearance of myself and which maintains my self.

Su Wen Chapter 5 is not a description of everything in the universe, it is a description of how man is constituted - so it starts from the direction, the location, which here is the central region, because that is the starting point of any individual. Then it comes to the first expression:

That which in Heaven makes dampness on Earth makes the soil or the Earth element.

地

土

This is equally true for me as for the universe, and if it is quoted here it is not to talk of Heaven or to talk of Earth, *di* , but to talk of dampness and to talk of soil, ie. the Earth element, *tu*. Not only the dampness you have outside, but the dampness you have inside, and not only the *tu,* the Earth as such, but the *tu* you have within yourself. Because you are really a crossing point of what makes Heaven Heaven and what makes Earth Earth.

When we want to know how a Chinese text is organized we have to look at the end, and from the end we have to come back to each of the pronouncements and relate them to the final sentences. When we say Heaven, Earth and Man it is not unusual for Man to be in the final position, it is normal to proceed from the start and come to the end. And that is very important because if we don't do that it's impossible for us to see how the text is coherent. In my opinion it is not a description of three powers, it is a description of the condition of Man.

That which in Heaven makes dampness, on Earth makes the Earth element, in the body makes the flesh.

This third part, *in the body makes flesh,* is the important point and relies on the two first pronouncements. In the following sentences 'that which' is implied although the character itself is not repeated. The governing character is *zai,* to be in among, no longer *sheng,* to produce. The *zai* character is used eleven times. The first six lines of this presentation used *sheng*, the seventh was *zhu,* to master and now what comes next? After the seventh character *zhu* what is the situation? The situation is that there is dampness. Now if I go on with this exploration of the condition of dampness then it no longer refers to Heaven but to Earth, and it will be the soil. Coming back to Ling Shu Chapter 8 we see that:

Heaven in me is virtue and Earth in me is Breath

so we understand that they are making some sort of division. There is virtue in Heaven, that is true, but what is there on Earth? On Earth there is the virtue of Heaven working through Earth. How can I speak of that? What new word can I coin for the occasion? It must be Breath. So Breath is the same thing as virtue, but seen not from the viewpoint of Heaven, because then it would have been virtue, but from the viewpoint of Earth. Why do I say that is the same thing? Because I know that Earth imitates Heaven, and Earthly Breaths are really a replica of Heavenly virtue. So now I understand that Heavenly virtue in me is virtue and dampness, and that the Earthly part of myself is the Breath and the soil. So there are Breaths inside the soil and I myself am some sort of ground or soil where there is the power of Earth which is the Breath of Earth given by Heaven but under the dominant organization of Earth. The coming together of Heaven and Earth is my body, and within my body what should I call it? I call it flesh.

Then we can come back to what we have been saying, that flesh is more a place for *qi,* which is under Heavenly virtue, and this is very consistent with the teaching of Zhuang Zi Chapter 2.

So why do they now go on to talk about the five *zang?* Because when man is built, in order to have the highest life for that organization and organism, a new word has to be coined, and the word is thesaurization or *zang.* The organs are *zang,* and the effect of these organs is thesaurization, *zang,* because there is no choice in the Chinese vocabulary to say whether *zang* is more the function or more the location where the function takes place. The life of man is exactly at the crossing of Heaven and Earth, so whatever has been said of Heaven and Earth has to be said of Man. The governing organs of the body are the *zang,* and at the level of the central region you call this particular *zang,* Spleen.

Then we go from one instance to another and we see that everything falls in line at the right place in this elaboration of the Spleen, and we have aspects, notes, sounds, and movements etc.

Elisabeth talked of the five instances of will which are not exactly wills as we understand it, because for us will is an intellectual process, but for the Chinese will is just an expression of life when it is rooted in the *zang.* We have to understand why they are talking of will here in connection with thinking, and how there is some sort of central position in their thinking, because everything has the connotation of the central region. Because Man occupies the Centre of the universe it is proper for him to be a thinker.

Also, because it is a medical book, we have to understand how all these Breaths can go astray and if they do, how we can compensate for it. This is given in those different items about how you can counteract the violence done by dampness, and what happens when the taste is not in equilibrium, and what is the difference between taste and dampness. Elisabeth was saying that if you are considering the air, or the sky, or Heaven, or the atmospheric agents, there is a place for the organization by five. But if you want to take all that inside the Earth where all the

60

products for your own assimilation are produced then you have to refer to the sweetness inside the taste, and that is something common between sweetness and dampness. It is quite obvious because Earth is just a replica of Heaven.

I want to stress the phenomenal brightness of the Chinese presentation in Chapter 5. Elisabeth and I have been doing a lot of work on this chapter in order to prepare a presentation of how Man is organized under the meeting of *yin* and *yang*, and the only way to see that is not to place Man outside the universe, but on the contrary to see how Heaven and Earth pour out their influences to make us come forth. That for me is the logic of the chapter.

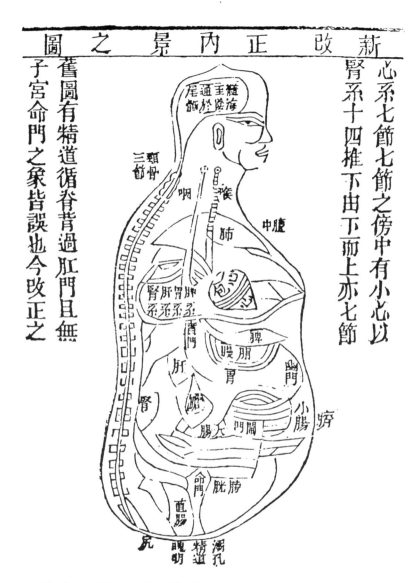

新改正內景之圖

心系七節七節之傍中有小心以
腎系十四椎下由下而上亦七節

舊圖有精道循脊背過肛門且無
子宮命門之象皆誤也今改正之

The Internal Organs from Yi Zong Pi Tu, compiled about 1575 AD

SU WEN CHAPTER 9

Elisabeth Rochat: Now we arrive at Su Wen Chapter 9. In this chapter there is a special place for the Stomach and Intestines.

The five Tastes penetrate by the mouth and are thesaurized in and by the Intestines and Stomach, and this thesaurization of the five Tastes is for the maintenance and nourishment of the five Breaths.

This expression 'the five Breaths' has the meaning of the Breaths of the five *zang.* They are the Breaths of life in the five aspects which support life. When the Breaths are in an harmonious composition you have life, the body liquids are perfectly balanced and the Spirits spontaneously make this man alive and are life itself.

Spleen, Stomach, Large Intestine, Small Intestine, Triple Heater, Bladder: these are the root of the storehouses and granaries, the dwelling place of nutrition. Its name is utensil.

There is possibility for transformation giving residues and dregs, for the transmission of the Tastes as well as the entries and exits.

至 陰

Its flourishing spect is in the four whites of the lips, the power of its fullness is in the flesh; its taste is sweet, its colour yellow. Its category is extreme yin, and it is in free communication with the Breaths of the Earth.

You know that we call the Stomach the Sea of the five *zang* and six *fu,* the Sea of Liquids and Cereals, the Sea of Breaths and so on. In Su Wen Chapter 9 we have this formation and enumeration of each of the five *zang* with a definition of what is fundamental and what kind of root for life each is able to be. Each *zang* is presented alone, with the Heart first, then Lung, Kidneys and Liver, and in the fifth position, Spleen. With the Spleen the *fu* are presented - not the six *fu,* but five of the six, the five which are the *fu* for transportation and transformation, the

傳化之府 *chuan hua zhi fu.* They are the Stomach, Large Intestine, Small

Intestine, Triple Heater and Bladder. The Gall Bladder is not a *fu* for transportation and transformation but a special *fu,* a *qi heng zhi fu,* an Extraordinary *fu* for actively storing Essences.

The two ideograms which account for the function of the Spleen are very close to *chuan hua.* The function of the Spleen is *yun hua. Hua* has the meaning of transformation, and *yun,* a kind of transportation. *Chuan* is something like the transmission from one to another, or the following on from one to another, whereas *yun* is more a kind of distribution, a sending out into every place.

Claude Larre: I would like to make a subtle differentiation between the character *yun* and the character *chuan,* since it seems that *yun* is the natural way that things transport themselves to where they are needed, and *chuan* is on a lower level because it's the coarse operation of transmitting from this place to that indefinitely. In *yun* there is a higher treatment of life, it's more Heavenly influx, which means everything is revolving in the best order because that is the will of Heaven. And transmitting, *chuan,* is more from hand to hand, from one place to another at a lesser level.

Elisabeth Rochat: Of course, the Spleen is a *zang* and here we have the distribution of the group of five *fu,* but something is analogous and through that we can understand why the Spleen is presented with the retinue of *fu.* They all share this ability to transform, to give movement, to distribute and transport, but the Spleen does so in the way of a *zang* and the others in the way of the *fu.* Of course the Spleen has the ability to distribute influx in the body up to the extremities of the limbs, through the flesh and so on, and to distribute all nutritive Elements and Essences in the shape of bodily liquids. The *fu* are for transmission, transportation and transformation of the half digested bolus of food, and the transmission is from one *fu* to another. The Spleen is for the elevation of the clear and pure, the *fu* are for the descending of the unclear. In this context the Spleen is the 'root of the storehouses and granaries', *cang lin* - with the double aspect of being able to receive and

64

to give. We find the same expression in Su Wen Chapter 8 as the common charge of Spleen and Stomach. Here in Su Wen 9, *cang lin* are the 'dwelling place of nutrition', *ying*. *Ying* is a special ideogram for that which we call nutritional Breaths.

Question: Or nutritive Breaths?

Elisabeth Rochat: Nutritive is maybe not enough because *ying* also has the meaning of building and rebuilding: renewing the constitution and structure: maintaining the shape of the body and nourishing all the elements.

Claude Larre: The problem is that *ying qi* is ready to use right now, everything is prepared and everything is ready for assimilation.Whereas nutritive Breaths are not prepared but can be used later for nourishment and nutrition. So it is a question of choosing between those two words. There is no activity if there is no nutrition, but it is only when all the nutritive processes have been completed that may you use whatever energy is then contained in your body after the transformation, and that's *ying qi*.

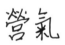

Elisabeth Rochat: These five *fu,* Stomach, Large intestine, Small Intestine, Triple Heater and Bladder are like storehouses and granaries for the body, receiving food, and through transformation participating in the task of nourishing the Essences and the *jing wei*. In another way they are also used for the elimination of waste, with the downward movement mastered by the Stomach. In this case Stomach is always at the beginning of the enumeration of the five *fu* of transmission and transformation because it is the first to receive food and it masters this movement of going down.

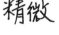

The Spleen is also like a storehouse and granary for the body, especially for the other *zang* and for the nutritive *ying* aspect of vitality. In this case the Spleen can distribute the nutritive influx and benefit the other *zang* and itself, by way of the five Tastes. With this movement of rising up of these very pure clear Breaths of nourishment and nutrition we have the idea of the double movement of Stomach and Spleen, ascending and descending. We can also see that the Spleen is the only *zang* which receives Essences of nutrition not yet completely divided up into five aspects, in the shape of the five Tastes for example, and the Spleen has the task of finishing this assimilation of Essences and distributing to each *zang* the taste of the quality of Essences which can be stored by that *zang,* and which renew that particular aspect of vitality. In this sense Spleen and Stomach are both storehouses and granaries, but each in its proper way, as *zang* or *fu.* Thus it is "the dwelling place of nutrition".

Its name is utensil, qi.

Claude Larre: This *qi* is a sort of vessel. It can be used for cooking, or when the food has been prepared it can be used to preserve the food. The ideogram shows four sections of bamboo - they are similar to the representation of mouths, but they are not mouths, they make the four feet of a sort of vessel which is used in order to make the cooking quicker - because it is able to come closer to the Fire. These four square figures, with this construction in the middle, are a very good representation of a vessel.

Elisabeth Rochat: This notion of a utensil goes well with what has been said about the meaning of Spleen, being like a servant, something able to help doing something. It's also the idea of cooking food in order to make it more assimilable. I think the meaning of utensil is also applicable to each of the five *fu* for transmission and transformation because they really are like utensils to the alimentation, and there is this interplay between the ascending and descending movement because when you cook you have evaporation and steam, and you also have something to throw away and something to keep which is good for the body. These kinds of ideas are all behind this ideogram.

There is possibility for transformation, hua, giving the residues and

66

dregs, zao po, for the transmission of the Tastes as well as the entries and exits, ru chu.

精微 The first result of transformation is *jing wei,* the transformation into Essences which are so subtle that they can become my Essences. But we have another part, at the end of the process there are the residues and dregs, the waste. The specific characteristics of residues and dregs are that they have no more Essences to be assimilated by the body, so they must go out of the body, and you know that when the Spleen is too weak you have the kind of diarrhoea in which residues and dregs are still full of Essences. It's a diarrhoea full of cereals, still with the pure and clear material of undigested food. We can see the link of Spleen with these evacuations and transformations, and the phenomenon of diarrhoea by the connection of the five *fu* with transmission and transformation.

The transmission of the Tastes is transmission of the five Essences, in the shape of the Tastes, to each *zang,* and the entries and exits are the two extremities of the process, the upper and lower orifices. All that is between these two openings is rooted in the Spleen and Stomach, with the Stomach mastering the Large Intestines, the Small Intestines, Triple Heater and Bladder.

魄 In Ling Shu Chapter 8, entries and exits are linked with the *po,* and the
太陰 *po* are linked with the Essences. The *po* are connected with the Lung, so it is another way to see the power of *tai yin* to give substantial form through transformation and entries and exits.

Its flourishing aspect , hua, is at the four whites of the lips.

The four whites of the lips are the four corners of the lips - it's quite interesting because it refers to the white flesh at the corners of the lips and in French or English I think we only mention two corners. But in Chinese we have four corners in order to see how, by the power of the Spleen, the flesh is well maintained and nourished in four directions. You also know that these two ideograms, *si bai,* are the name of a very
四白 important point [Stomach 2]. The name of Spleen 3 is *tai bai* which is
太白

the great white of great whites. Some Chinese commentaries make a connection between these two expressions. The lips are a mark of the prosperity of the Spleen because the lips are a more manifest, more external form of flesh, and flesh is just the movement of the Spleen in the body at the level of the structure of the body.

Claude Larre: One point might be to understand why they talk of white, because white has two opposite meanings. One is the lack of life associated with a deceased person or the colour for funerals, and the other is the sparkling sunny quality of light. Sunny light is understood because the character is made by the radical for sun with a stroke on top. Since there are two lips and four *bai* it's necessary that the brightness should be seen on the face and on the body itself. What is important is that the Fire of life can really be seen. The brightness is the effect of the Essences. While the Essences are hidden, they are thesaurized and they are *zang*. But because we have Essences we maintain them and therefore the Spirits have a good place to be, and that is actually what we can see through the body. Everything which is well organized and full of strength in the internal structure, has to be shown outside, and it has to be shown in the bodily place where function appears. The function of Spleen has to do with the renewal of the body, and life to renew the body through alimentation comes at the mouth. So it's in the four corners there that we can see whether everything is in order in the relation between Spleen and Stomach. We can see the same thing with the Heart; the place to see whether the Heart is really peaceful and void is on the face. We know that the Liver is the power of life in the ascent, like Spring and the vital impulse, and we know that for the Chinese the eyes are the way to accept images and send messages, so the message of life of the Liver is seen in the clarity and brightness of the eye.

The character for appearance and for body is the same, *xing*. When we write *xing* we translate it body, shape or external shape. We are now sure that in the embryo there is no shape, but there is full life. And at death there is no more life, but only shape. So it's absolutely vital to understand that *biao li* or *yin yang* are internal qualities manifesting externally. Life is always inside, in the middle and in the obscurity, but

68

it will always be showing itself. That is the deepest consideration of what life might be, it's the way for Earth to receive Heaven and to produce a being in which Heaven and Earth will be showing their relationship. And this has to be seen for the Heart, for Liver, for Spleen and all the rest.

So the teaching is always current and is always analogous, and what we have to do one year to another is to simplify all the problems that we get from teaching acupuncture in the Western way, or even of the teaching of the Chinese books themselves. Because if they are repetitious it's just the passing of time which obliges people to write something about something which is already so clear and simple in itself! It's something to live with, it's not something to explain.

Elisabeth Rochat:

The power of its fullness is in the flesh; its taste is sweet; its colour yellow. Its category is extreme yin and it is in free communication with the Breaths of the Earth.

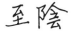

Some commentators say that the Spleen is *zhi yin,* extreme *yin,* because all things return to the Earth, and return to the soil, so the Spleen is the greatest *yin* because it can receive all kinds of things. This is the end and beginning of the process of nourishment, maintenance and distribution of life.

..it is in free communication with the Breaths of the Earth.

The Spleen is in free communication with the Breaths of the Earth unlike the other *zang* which are in free communication with the Breaths of one of the four seasons. There is no representation of a fifth season. But we'll see in Su Wen Chapter 29 what the meaning of that is and what time or moment is ruled by the Spleen.

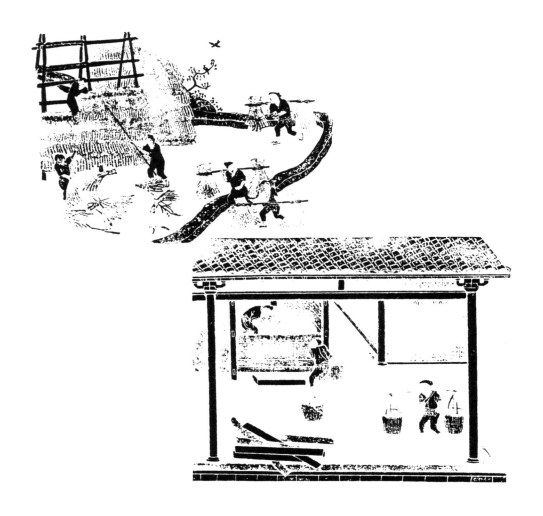

Storehouses and Granaries, *cang lin*

SU WEN CHAPTER 11

Fullness and emptiness in the *zang fu*

In Su Wen Chapter 11 there is a very clear differentiation between *zang* and *fu,* and I will spend some minutes explaining that, because there was a question about it this morning. The question was that if we see in certain books that *yin* is void or empty and *yang* is fullness, how can you explain that *yin* can be either full or empty? The answer is in Su Wen Chapter 11. It's very simple in Chinese, but a little bit complicated in English.

The five zang actively thesaurize jing qi

You know these two ideograms *jing qi,* Essences and Breaths. Remember, it's important not to say Essential Breaths - but something like Essences/Breaths or Essences and Breaths as *jing qi* are Essences stored actively by each *zang* in order to allow the releasing of *qi.* The *zang* don't allow the Essences to seep away because *jing qi,* Essences/Breaths, are the foundation of vitality, and there is no reason why these very choice, pure Breaths realized from Essences should have to go outside . If they did it would mean loss of life. For this reason we see the *zang* are full of *man* fullness, and they cannot be full with *shi* fullness. The meaning of these two ideograms, *man,* and *shi,* is fullness, but in two different ways. *Man* is like an impregnation - very subtle. At this level *zang* can be *man* because they are completely impregnated with Essences and Breaths, all very clear and pure and with the support of the Spirits and so on.

Conversely, the six *fu* are for transmission and transformation, *chuan hua,* and for this reason they are unable to keep and store. So they are *shi* and they can't be *man* because they receive something and then they act by transforming and afterwards transmitting. They are *shi* when they contain food or when food is engaged in the process of digestion. For example, when the Stomach receives food and transforms and ferments it, the Stomach is said to be full, *shi*. Afterwards, when the Stomach transmits the remainder of the food to the Small Intestine, the Stomach is empty. It's just waiting for the next meal. But *zang* always have to be in a *man* state of fullness, it's not possible for a *zang* to be empty. This is the way that the *yin zang* are full in the body, and the way in which the *yang fu* are full in the body and it's not the same way. It's impossible to say *yin* is void or *yang* is in fullness. The way of being empty or full is not the same for *yin* and *yang*, or *zang* and *fu*, but because nothing on Earth is purely *yin* or *yang*, everything is composed of Elements and the important point is to have a good balance of *yin* and *yang* according to the special nature of each species.

Question: You spoke before of nutriments which had not yet assumed the identity of the person, would you require *zang* to store *man* substances which had acquired that identity?

Elisabeth Rochat: I think the guarantee for this identity are the Kidneys and the Essences of the Kidneys and Anterior Heaven. The Essences of Anterior Heaven are not merely Essences which are present at the moment of conception. They are the inborn mechanism and structure for the rebuilding and reconstitution of the body on the model of the first composition of the two Essences of the father and mother, a proper meeting or joining of Fire and Water, *yin* and *yang* and so on. The Kidneys are the guarantee for this, and this function is the meaning of the Essences of the Kidneys. If the Essences of the Kidneys are deficient or weak then there is a lack of these Essences and linked to such a weakness of the Kidneys we have all the deformities of childhood. The Breaths of the Spleen are said to be the Trunk of Posterior Heaven, and the Breaths of the Kidneys to be the Trunk of Anterior Heaven. Both are necessary for the maintenance and nourishment of an individual life, along with respiration. So we have the three feminine *zang,* Lung, Spleen and Kidneys working on the Essences. We can also see this in Su Wen Chapter 21.

The Stomach as Sea of Liquids and Cereals

In Su Wen Chapter 11 we see that:

The Stomach is the Sea of liquids and cereals

This is the first important mention of the Stomach set apart from the other *fu*. In general the Stomach appears a lot more than the other *fu* because it has a more important function. Chapter 11 is a good example because here the Stomach has a special presentation with this definition of being a 'Sea of liquids and cereals' - and we remember that the Stomach is one of the four seas of the body along with *tan zhong* (Sea of Breaths), the brain (Sea of Marrow), and *chong mai* (Sea of Blood).

膻中
衝脈

The Stomach is the great gushing source from which springs out all that is necessary for the maintenance of the six *fu*.

The five Tastes enter the mouth and are stored in the Stomach to maintain the Breaths of the five zang.

We can see that in Su Wen Chapter 11 there is a contradiction because at the beginning of the chapter it says that the six *fu* are unable to thesaurize or store, but now we read that the five Tastes are stored in the Stomach. It's difficult to understand, but it's because the Chinese language is very strict and very flexible at the same time. The meaning is that if you see the Stomach as the source of the maintenance of the five *zang*, which are active places for the realizing of Breaths, you are speaking of Essences and Breaths, and if you are speaking of Essences and Breaths you are speaking of what must be necessarily kept inside the body for its vitality. So for this reason you use the ideogram to store. The Stomach is not only one of the six *fu* for transmission and transforming, but it is also the main place for the extraction of Essences and for the realizing of Breaths through the five *zang*. For this reason, in other chapters of the Su Wen and Ling Shu we have the Stomach described as the Sea of the five *zang* and six *fu*. For example in Su Wen Chapter 34 and Ling Shu Chapter 29 you can see this double

脾胃論 aspect of the Stomach. This is a good quotation from which to grasp the particular importance and place of the Stomach in old Chinese texts and in Chinese medicine. A very famous treatise on the Spleen and Stomach, Pi Wei Lun, was written in the 12th century AD. It deals with most diseases in relation to the Spleen and Stomach and it's a very interesting book.

Su Wen Chapter 11 continues by saying:

The mouth of Breaths is tai yin, therefore Breaths and Tastes of the five zang and six fu all come from the Stomach and their alterations are visible at the mouth of the Breaths.

Mouth of Breaths is the name for the pulses, it means a mouth like an opening or passage, a way by which you can reach the Breaths. Most of the time it designates the radial pulse. You can see here the connection and compenetration of *yin* and *yang* through *zang* and *fu* and through the Breaths and Tastes, and everything is said to come from the power of the Stomach as the main place for this reconstitution of life. We also have this idea that the Stomach and Spleen have a very close connection. They share the same function, granaries and storehouses and so on, and 精微 they act together to produce and transport bodily liquids and *jing wei*. You also know that the Breaths of *tai yin* of the foot, Spleen, rise up to 宗氣 the Sea of Breaths in the Upper Heater to join with the quintessence of respiration in order to form the Ancestral Breaths, the *zong qi*.

Another point made in this text is that Spleen is very close to Stomach, and we see that it's by Stomach, and Spleen acting as a helper to the Stomach, that the five *zang* and six *fu* can remain alive and in activity and can fulfill their tasks. In this case it's because of the Stomach and the Breaths of the Stomach that the *zang* and *fu* are in good or bad form and you can see that through the meridian of *Tai Yin* of the hand at the Mouth of Breaths.

This same idea is given in Su Wen Chapter 18:

稟 *The normal Breaths of the well-balanced man are received, lin, from the*

Stomach. The Stomach is the normal Breaths of the well balanced man. When a man no longer has the Breaths of the Stomach then it is called "counter-current", and this counter-current is death.

This *lin* is very close to the *lin* which has the meaning of granaries. The meaning is very simple. Each zang and fu and each meridian needs the Breaths of the Stomach to remain in activity. And as it is said here, if you don't eat for one or two days your pulse first appears disturbed and you grow weaker and weaker, and then after some time you die. It's a countercurrent of the norm of life which is to eat two or three times a day. For us it's not a normal problem, but it was at that time, and still is now for a lot of people.

It's very simple: if you want to remain alive you have to breathe and eat, and you have to have good transformation, assimilation and elimination. Of course, you have to have all these functions at different levels of your life, for food and for respiration, and if they are well regulated and your brain and your Spirit are very clear then you can eliminate all the bad waste and dregs, and also bad ideas and thoughts. It's the same movement. You can see that if you have patients with Spleen and Stomach pathology, they are very often bloated or have some problem with diarrhoea or constipation. At the same time they often have a problem with mental elimination.

Later in Su Wen Chapter 18 there is a presentation of the pulse of each *zang* in relationship to the power of the Breaths of the Stomach.

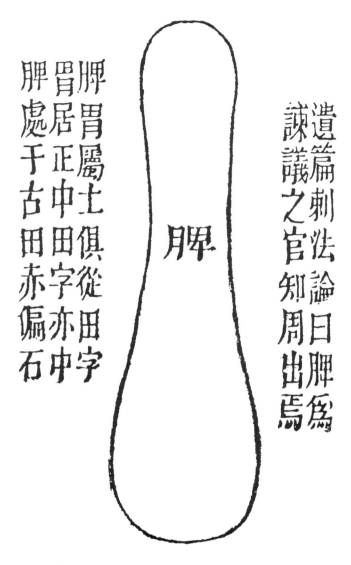

脾胃屬土俱從田字
胃居正中田字亦中
脾處于古田赤偏石

遺篇刺法論曰脾爲
諫議之官知周出焉

The Spleen from the Ling Shu Su Wen Jie Yao

76

THE SPLEEN

Su Wen Chapter 23

Elisabeth Rochat: We will now see some complementary information on the Spleen from the Nei Jing. Su Wen Chapter 23 presents the special function of each *zang* and *fu* in relation to the five Tastes, the five Breaths, the five emotions and so on. It discusses the places where the five Tastes enter, acid enters the Liver, sweet enters the Spleen and so on, and from the pathological point of view the place where the Breaths of the five *zang* become ill. The Spleen, for example, makes regurgitations, and in this case especially acid regurgitations. The explanation of this is that the Spleen helps the Stomach to make a good circulation of bodily liquids, but when the Breaths of the Spleen are weak and ill they can no longer water and humidify the *zang,* and therefore bodily liquids cannot be distributed in the four directions or to the four *zang,* so they move in a countercurrent to the mouth and the pharynx, and you have this kind of regurgitation. Most of the time these regurgitations are acid because it is a movement of Wood against Earth, Gall Bladder and Liver against Spleen and Stomach.

The Spleen fears dampness because it is rooted in soil and dampness, and for that reason likes dryness, although not too dry. Spleen fears the extreme dampness because, as we saw, dampness provokes a loosening of the circulation and this loosening implies some blockage in circulation. You know that dampness oppresses or embarrasses the circulation of the Breaths of the Spleen. In this case the Spleen can no longer fulfill its task to transport, to distribute and to transform. At the level of the flesh dampness makes flaccidity and oedema and so on.

On the other hand, the Stomach fears dryness because of its own nature, Stomach needs humidity, dampness, and liquids in order to make its fermentation, maceration and transformation.

In another part of Su Wen Chapter 23 it says that Spleen is or makes saliva. In the same context Kidneys are or make spittle. I think the difference between saliva and spittle is that spit is to go outside the body, but saliva is to remain in the mouth to allow good functioning of the tongue and the mouth, to begin the digestion and all that process, and to allow the tongue to move and speak.

Afterwards we have some sentences that you already know:

意

Spleen thesaurizes yi
Spleen masters the flesh

In this way, in the relationship between Spleen and flesh we can see that the deepness and density of the Earth is an exact analogy with the thickness and density of the flesh. Finally in relation to the *mai* or *mo*, the network and current of animation, or the pulses - the same word in Chinese, because the pulses are just a specific place where we can appreciate the quality of the current of animation - you know that each *zang* has a specific quality of the *mai* and the pulse of the Spleen is intermittent. Commentaries say that it is intermittent because this is a sign that you are passing from one season to another, that it's a sign of the succession of Breaths, or the twenty four different climatic periods of the year. The meaning of intermittent is just a little pause in order to pass on to another quality of Breaths. With this notion of succession or intermittence we have the idea of harmonization and well-tempered things. If the successions or passages are well done, all is well tempered and harmonized - there's an harmonious composition.

脉

Let me just recall Ling Shu Chapter 8. It talks of the mastering of Spleen over the *yi,* the purpose, and of all pathological aspects of that, when the Spleen is seized by melancholia and affliction. When we are unable to get rid of this oppression and trouble, the *yi,* the purpose, is injured, and when the *yi* is injured you can guess it will be the contrary of having an harmonious composition, the text says all is in disorder, perturbation and disturbance.

意

Claude Larre: One major teaching in Lao Zi is that the saintly kings of old had no fixed mind themselves but were complying with the changes of mind of their people. We know at the same time that the Heart has to be empty. If the Heart is empty and if the will is constant, it does not mean that the mind will not be subjected to so many images or ideas, and will not have the ability to change in order to adapt to any different circumstances.

So there is a difference between being able to adapt to circumstances and getting into disorder with your purpose. They are not the same thing. They look as if they are the same thing because everything looks like changing. It's not that everything is changing, but that you have the ability to change if it is necessary in order to adapt yourself to certain conditions. We know that this is really an excellent thing and something that the Chinese can do very easily. But how is it possible that they are always on the verge of change? In fact you see that they are not changing so much, and that they are still the dominating power, so life has been understood by them as something to which you have to adapt because it is always in constant change. When Ling Shu Chapter 8 stresses that under the influence of oppression and sorrow, purpose is no longer stable, it does not mean that previously it was fixed in stability, it means that the condition of determination has to be there even if you change every moment. You change because you want to change. It is not the same thing as not being able to keep your own will, purpose, or the like. So diseases are when those changes are made outside your will, or outside your purpose. This point is very clear in the Chinese philosophy of life but not so clear with us, because when somebody changes we say, "Ah, you changed". And all the critics of the person ask, "Why did you change?"

Elisabeth Rochat: At the same time as this deep disorder in the interior functioning of the body happens, because the Spleen can no longer be the turntable and place for all permutations and harmonization, the four limbs cannot move, the hair on the skin gets brittle, you have signs of premature death and you die during the Spring. This is because Spring is the period during the year when the natural impulse is to go far away and to rise up powerfully and so on, and if inside your intimate reaction,

action and functioning you are oppressed and blocked at the level of the Spleen, it's impossible for you to have this kind of rising up during the Spring. You have something similar at the end of Ling Shu Chapter 8 in this quotation:

Spleen thesaurizes ying, (ying as in nutritive, rebuilding power)
and ying is the dwelling place of the yi.

This is quite important because between nutrition, *ying,* and what we call *yi,* there is a mutual connection of effect. *Yi* needs some support in order to manifest itself as efficient, and *ying* cannot be efficient if it is not inhabited by one of the five highest entities of life.

When the Breaths of the Spleen are empty or on the way to becoming empty, the four limbs cannot be used.

Claude Larre: It's not only that you can't use them, they don't want to be used. You never know where your consciousness is in your body. It's too easy to say I have in the heart of my Heart the purpose to live. The trouble is that we have four limbs, and those four limbs want to live, but they accept to live in obedience to and at the service of all the body. Yet it might be that there is a limb which doesn't want to give service and there is a revolt in the organization. So it seems to be a very Westernized point of view to say that everything is under the Heart or the Lungs, for example, they are all servants in turn and maybe one of them is lord at a certain time. Of course, all that is under the supervision, authority and sovereignty of the big three, Heart, Lung and Liver. But it would be good to represent life not only in the headquarters but everywhere, as in a country. Maybe the government is the governing agent but there are many citizens, and some of them may group themselves together and may revolt against the central authority. It could be the same in an individual. It might be that the limbs don't want to move because they can't. So it might be safer to be very strict with the translation and say that the four limbs don't want to.

80

Elisabeth Rochat: In the light of this text, in connection with the *ying,* nutritive power, and *yi ,* we can see that the four limbs are no longer used because they are not nourished, irrigated or watered by the Spleen, and also because the *yi* can no longer rise and give the idea of moving these limbs to the Spirits. It's exactly like the Empire - if the central government is weak, the maintenance, the army, the soldiers and all kinds of transportation cannot arrive at the borders or frontiers, and the orders from the government don't arrive either. Worst still, perhaps they are not even very well organized at the Centre of government, because the government no longer knows where it is going and there is no correct or well-formulated order. We have this situation in every state at some time during history. Everything becomes mixed and confused because of this central weakness.

Claude Larre: This expression "four limbs" is seen everywhere in the text, it means hands and feet, but it also means all external activity, in contrast to all the nutrition and internal activities. So when they say the four limbs won't move it doesn't only mean that the hands and feet are no longer usable, it means that everything manifesting externally is ceasing to function. This is the problem with schizophrenia or anorexia and things like that, when there is some sort of slow immobilization and you cannot reach the mind of the person, and at the same time you see that there is no external activity. If you cannot get to the mind of the person and at the same time you see no external activity, maybe the fact is that the *yi* is no longer functioning. So if you talk to the person, because there is no *yi* there is no place for purpose and no way for them to understand what you are saying. There is no reason for a disruption in the organization externally, unless internally something is so much in disorder that it is no longer functioning. We are not supposed to separate the external motion from the inner organization because we know that the external motion is just the manifestation of the condition of the inner structure, where the *zang,* the *yi,* the *zhi,* the Spirits and all of that are making life.

Elisabeth Rochat: At the same time as the four limbs are out of use or order, the five *zang* are no longer peaceful. We can see that if the five *zang* are peaceful, there are good relationships between them, and on the contrary, if the relationships are bad and there is no regularization between the *zang,* it's because the Spleen's Breaths are empty. When Spleen's Breaths are full, (ie. when the fullness is not a good fullness but a perversion, such as a blockage or obstruction) the Stomach is swollen and all the transmissions that can take place in the lower part of the abdomen are blocked. This could be seen in micturation, in stools or in menstruation for women.

Ling Shu Chapter 29

In Ling Shu Chapter 29 we have quite an interesting quotation which says that the Spleen is very active in the defence of the organism.

The Spleen, its mastership is defence.

精微

The explanation of this sentence in the classical commentaries is that because the Spleen has mastery over distribution and transformation it is able to distribute Essences from the *jing wei* to any part of the body and especially to the five *zang,* and the four limbs, which as Father Larre has said, means any part of the body with exterior activity. By this work, the Spleen makes the power and strength of man's defence particularly against attacks coming from the exterior.

Su Wen Chapter 52

Another description appears in Su Wen Chapter 52:

使 市

The Spleen is the messenger, shi, the Stomach is the market, shi.

You see that the Chinese play very easily with words, homophones and

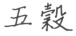

so on, *shi* and *shi*. We also see this messenger character, *shi* , when studying the Heart and the Heart as Master. It means a messenger and an agent by which something can be done. A commentator says, a messenger is a man or person who goes far away and who makes things known - like an ambassador. The Spleen masters transportation, distribution and transformation of liquids and cereals to nourish and maintain all parts of the body. In this way the Spleen is messenger because it can circulate the Breaths of cereals in order to maintain every part of the body and the *zang*.

The Stomach is like a market because it receives the five cereals and helps with the transmission of the Breaths of the Spleen to nourish the five *zang*. It is like a market, a place of commerce or a fairground, where merchants bring things and sell them, and other people leave the market with the things they've sold. It's a place for exchange, for transformation or transportation. It's also the place where all things can be gathered to be exchanged or to participate in the maintenance of life for each family, each person and so on. And to be a market has a resemblance to being a sea.

Ling Shu Chapter 17

When the Breaths of the Spleen are in free communication with the mouth, the Spleen is in harmony and the mouth can distinguish the five cereals, wu gu.

Elisabeth Rochat: The meaning is that through the Breaths of the Spleen, through their good state and harmonization, we are able to recognize what food we have in our mouth, and we can distinguish and know the five cereals. In this chapter of the Ling Shu it is by the activity and action of the Breaths of the Heart that you can distinguish the five Tastes. It's exactly as if the Tastes were the inner structure of food, and you need the Breaths of the Heart to penetrate to the interior of another thing. But through the Spleen and the Breaths of the Spleen you can recognize what kind of food you have in your mouth. This is not exactly the same thing. Of course you know that one of the most important symptoms of the Spleen is lack of taste or disturbance in the taste, but I think that this is more the immediate taste not so much this ability of the Heart to penetrate to the intimate structure of another thing. And in the context of this chapter the Spleen is said to distinguish the five cereals, the Heart the five Tastes.

Ling Shu Chapter 43

When the Breaths of the Spleen rise in power, one dreams of singing and music and that the body is heavy and can no longer move.

When the weakening Breaths are the hosts of the Spleen, in dreaming one sees mounds and hills and great marshes; one dreams that the house is ruined by wind and rain.

Elisabeth Rochat: Ling Shu Chapter 43 has to do with the meaning of dreams. It is very easy to see that this kind of joyful singing is the proper expression of the Spleen and the Earth and the central region, and that when we have the rising power of the Breaths of the Spleen we have the expression of this kind of sound when dreaming. At the same time you dream that the body is heavy and can no longer move because there is too great an abundance of the Spleen's Breaths in the flesh.

The weakening Breaths refers to the introduction of perverse energies by counter-current, following a deficiency of normal Breaths. This second part is quite interesting. Why do we see mounds and hills and great marshes? It's because the Spleen is the dwelling place of the *ying,* nutritive power, and the Spleen is like a utensil and must have flesh to shape the body, so when these kinds of Breaths are empty or too weak you have an emptiness on the Earth, and as a result an overflowing of Water. You just see the eroded part of the Earth in the form of mounds and hills and you dream at the same time of hills and mounds and great marshes. Marshes are exactly like Water invading Earth or soil. And the humidity and dampness are too strong like the Water in the reverse *ke* cycle. We saw yesterday that Spleen can also be considered as the image of the Earth, or like a house where everything in the body can be as if at home. So we dream that the house is ruined by wind and rain. Wind and Water are the two most important internal agents of perturbation for the Spleen. And for the Stomach:

When the weakening Breaths are the hosts of the Stomach one dreams of drinking and eating.

There is no need for commentary.

Claude Larre: The question is why do they attach so much importance to dreams? Usually we forget them because they are not real life. But for a Chinese expert life is equally real during dreams as during the time when you are not dreaming, and dreams must have their bearing or their point.

I remember when I was in Japan I happened to go and visit a temple and there was a special place for the rectification of dreams. The monks would go to the dispensary and be given herbs to correct the imbalance shown in their dreams. As far as I can understand it the imaginary power has a free release during the time we are lying in bed, but free as it might be it has to follow one direction or another. It has to follow a source of dreams, and those dreams, even if they are free, are more or less under the control of the five *zang,* because the *hun* and the *zang* are so intimately connected that the *zang* would give the *hun* one direction or another.

Question: When you say rectification of dreams do you mean an explanation?

Claude Larre: No, no. I said it was a dispensary. When you go to a dispensary it is to be cured. It doesn't mean that every morning everybody goes and corrects their dreams, but it was a Buddhist temple, and we know that Buddhists have a much more refined understanding of how to use psychology than anyone else. Before there were Buddhist monks in China the Chinese had dreams and perhaps they were interpreting dreams, but they didn't have an institution for it, it was left for everybody to do. But since the arrival of the Buddhists, Chinese spiritual life has become much more organized. The reason the Chinese government does not like the Buddhists or the Daoists is just because they are dealing with the conscience and with intellectual power. I don't talk of Christians because the Christian doesn't usually care about those details. The Chinese government doesn't like the Christians because of their connection with the powers outside China, not because they are harmful for the country, but they look very closely at the Daoists and the Buddhists.

Su Wen Chapter 22

When the Spleen is ill, the body is heavy. One is easily hungry, the flesh is flaccid (without power, impotent), the feet cannot receive and walk properly; when one walks one easily gets cramps. One has pain in the lower part of the leg. In case of emptiness the abdomen is congested and the intestines gurgle, one has diarrhoea where food has not been digested, one takes (needles) the meridians concerned, tai yin and yang ming as well as shao yin, bled.

Elisabeth Rochat: This is just in order to point out the connection between Spleen and Stomach and Kidneys, which is quite exceptional to this presentation of Su Wen Chapter 22 - it's not only *tai yin* and *yang ming* that are needled, but *shao Yin* of the foot, the meridian of the Kidneys. For the symptoms there is no problem in interpretation, but it is very important to see the connection between the Kidneys and the Water of the Kidneys, and the Spleen and the dampness of the Spleen - just as the origin of the power of nutrition and defence, of Breaths and

Blood and the power and strength of origin are in the Kidneys and by the Kidneys and through the Kidneys. The renewal of nutrition and defence, Blood and Breaths, and so on is made through the activity of the Spleen and Stomach - and that is the reason why in order to restore the free communication of Breaths in the meridians you treat with these three meridians, *tai yin* and *yang ming,* but also *shao yin.* Sometimes commentaries indicate points such as Spleen 5 to disperse the fullness of the Spleen, or Stomach 41, the tonification point of the Stomach, and Kidney 7, the tonification point for Kidneys. The treatment is done on the lower parts of the body because you are trying to disperse the congestion which is in the lower part of the trunk. All this was just to see that the connection between the Spleen and Kidneys is sometimes very important in treatment.

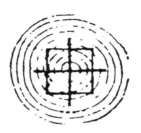

Biao li relationship of Spleen and Stomach

Elisabeth Rochat: Now we can look at a very important chapter, Su Wen Chapter 29. The title of the chapter is *Tai Yin Yang Ming*, and the chapter deals with Spleen and Stomach and the relationship between them.

黄帝
太陰
陽明
表裏

Huang Di said, tai yin and yang ming have a biao li relationship

...this is not an internal external relationship, a *biao li* relationship is a movement which allows the connections between internal and external, and that's not exactly the same.

Claude Larre: The *biao li* is the go-between. By internal you mean the part of you which is so much your heaven-self that you have no access to it, and external means the nice physical appearance we all have and everything connected with it, a house, a garden, the world and all that. Something to be seen and to be used. It doesn't mean that there is an inner space and an outer space. The answer is to dismiss the question of space and say that everything which is described in space has something to do with external, and everything which has nothing to do in itself with space is called internal. But since there is no internal except for the external, and no external except for the internal, there must be some connection between the one and the other. The connection is just that what cannot be seen becomes visible not by itself but by means of the external, and the foundation of the external lies in the invisible. This is the reason why they have *biao* and *li*, since *biao* is to manifest and *li* is to be such that the manifestation will be different. For each *li* there is *biao*, and for each *biao* there must be a fundamental *li*. And the *biao li* is the to and fro for the *nei* and *wai* (inner and outer).

内外
陰陽

With this sort of explanation we can understand that something very similar in Heaven and Earth and *yin* and *yang* is used for *nei wai* and *biao li*. Then Heaven Earth is the ultimate reality which is coming out unceasingly from the chaos. When I say coming out it doesn't mean that it's not in the chaos, but it might be seen outside the chaos while still being in the chaos. All the phenomena of life cannot exist and are not intelligible except through the *yin yang* device. The Chinese were keen enough on the subject to make two for one and one for two, they had one, the chaos, and inside the chaos they had this distinction between Heaven and Earth, but for the movement of Heaven towards Earth and the obedience of Earth towards Heaven they had to find an expression, and the expression they found is *yin yang*. Not that Earth is purely *yin* and Heaven purely *yang*, but by appropriation the closest to Heaven is *yang* and the closest to Earth is *yin*. In order that everything is on the move it is necessary that the virtue of Heaven has an aspect of *yin*, so the virtue of Heaven is *yin* and *yang*, but the initiative for the productivity is on the *yang* side and the effectiveness of this productivity relies upon the *yin* aspect of Heavenly virtue.

Elisabeth Rochat: When you say that *tai yin* and *yang ming* are in a *biao li* relationship the meaning is that inside the Earth Element there exists a two-fold possibility of going to the exterior or going to the interior. This is in a normal state and also in a pathological state, because perverse Breaths can follow the way of orthodox Breaths. But why do these two meridians and two viscera which represent the same Element produce such different illnesses?

Qi Bo answers:

Yin and yang have different locations, they are by turns, one after the other, empty and full, one after the other going against the current and going with the current. Their source is not the same, and this is why their illnesses have different names.

This is quite difficult to understand, but the meaning is very rich. The first differentiation is between *yin* and *yang* and by this we can see that Spleen and Stomach are like *yin* and *yang* beating together. For this reason they share a common charge in Su Wen Chapter 8. There is a prototype of the division and the beating in the dialectics of *yin yang*. Because they are so close, they are also very different and must be differentiated very carefully, as Father Larre said earlier in relation to Liver and Gall Bladder, they are so close and yet so far apart.

So what is the meaning of these different sites or locations? One is *yin* and has its mastering in the lower part, one is *yang* and has its mastering in the upper part. That is completely different to this movement of ascending and descending, but we'll see that in a little while. The dialectics and the assonance between the two, *yin* and *yang*, Spleen and Stomach, are the basic principle of their activity. Also, they share in the totality of life in the organism or in the harmonization of the intimate Breaths of my body with the external cosmos. This is because this kind of movement from empty to full and so on, one after the other, with or against the current, can also deal with the succession of seasons according to a lot of commentaries. During two seasons, Spring and Summer, *yang* is ascending, and during the other two seasons, Autumn and Winter, *yin* is ascending and *yang* descending. In the body, Spleen and Stomach are really the prototype of this succession, this alternating, and this complementary ascending and descending of *yin* and *yang*.

We saw in Chapter 11 that from the work of the Spleen and Stomach the *zang* and *fu* can obtain all that they need to live and remain in activity. Therefore, the twelve meridians need the Breaths of the Stomach and the activity of the Stomach and Spleen to circulate, to exist, to be and to remain rich in Breaths and Blood. Blood needs the Essences of Spleen in order to be produced, renewed and rebuilt. We will see later in Su Wen Chapter 21 how we need the Breaths of the Stomach, through liquid and solid alimentation, to restore in us our animation.

For this reason, Spleen and Stomach, *yin* and *yang*, animation, maintenance, building and so on are the basis of the constitution and rebuilding of the twelve meridians. And this double movement is also manifested through the twelve meridians with their twelve centripetal and centrifugal movements. It's also the movement of clear and unclear, of what is very dense and rich and animated by a *yin* movement to be concentrated in the interior, to be centripetal, or being animated by a

Heavenly movement, in the image of *yang,* to be centrifugal. For example, centripetal vitality could be Essences joining *zang,* and the centrifugal vitality could be the clear *yang,* going out to the four limbs in order to make defence and animation and so on. But there are a lot of possible examples.

津

Some commentaries say the Spleen has a special mastery of *yin* meridians with their centrifugal movement, and that Stomach has a special mastering of *yang* meridians with their centripetal current. But why are these *yin* meridians animated by a centrifugal movement proper to the *yang?* For example, in the bodily liquids the *yang* part, the *jin,* is animated by a centrifugal movement. The explanation is exactly the same as in the case of the Spleen mastering ascending and the Stomach mastering descending movement. It is very simple. If you want to be in relationships, you have to be between *yin* and *yang* and between Heaven and Earth, and between all the terms of dual expression of a couple. Each thing keeps within its own nature something of the other half of the couple. For example, there is enough *yin* in the power of Heaven to make rain descend, and there is enough *yang* in the bosom of the Earth to make humidity and dampness rise up and form the clouds. The only way for Heaven and Earth to be in connection is for the influx of Heaven to descend and the influx of Earth to ascend - and if not it is impossible to have life. If Spleen and Stomach or *yin* and *yang,* or any dual expression of a couple or something in a dialectic relationship, are in the pattern of the model of Heaven and Earth we always have the repetition of the same movement. For this reason the Stomach masters descending movement and the Spleen masters ascending movement and a *yin* meridian can manifest *yin* power to have contact with *yang* by a centrifugal movement.

陰陽

老子

Claude Larre: This is clearly stated in Lao Zi Chapter 2 when it says that what is on high and what is low turn towards one another - so this is really more than a medical statement - we know that if it is in Lao Zi it is central to the Chinese view of reality.

Elisabeth Rochat: In this paragraph we have the mastery of Spleen and Stomach over the four seasons and the three *yin* and *yang* currents. This is through the four limbs which are also under the mastery or sovereignty of the Spleen and Stomach and the Earth Element and which are, in the human body, in the shape and manner of the four seasons of the year. This is an idea which is written about in the commentaries on the chapter and in many other texts, because this same division into four is an expression of the differentiation of Breaths. In time there are four seasons of the year and in the human body there is the animation of *yin* and *yang* in the four limbs. There is also the idea that Spleen and Stomach are like *yin* and *yang* and Heaven and Earth in a great complementary relationship.

And the Emperor said: *I would like to know these differences that you say exist between the illnesses of Spleen and Stomach.*

Qi Bo said: *The yang is the Breath of Heaven and it commands the exterior, and the yin is the Breath of Earth and it commands the interior. And thus the Dao or the normal way of yang is fullness, and the Dao or the normal way of yin is emptiness.*

What is the meaning of that? It's very simple, it's a question of pathological aggression. *Yang* masters the exterior, *yang* makes defence and the movement of defence against, particularly, perversity coming from the exterior. For this reason the way of *yang* is to be full of power and strength to resist external aggression, but if you yield to this aggression you will have a perverse fullness in the exterior. This is invasion of perverse Breaths leading to perverse fullness. On the other hand the power of *yin* is emptiness, but it can also be full of Essences, Breaths and vitality. The perversion of that is weakness and internal deficiency.

For this reason when you are attacked by robber winds, the perversities which profit by this emptiness - for example if there is a deficiency in the defence of the body - then it's the yang that receives them; when the solid and liquid foods are disturbed or if activity and rest are not given adequate time then it's the yin that receives this attack.

You can see that the *yang* receives attack from external agents of disease, and the *yin* receives internal agents of disease in the form of disturbance in alimentation. Fatigue and exhaustion also affect the *yin*. When the *yang* receives an attack it enters the six *fu,* and when the yin receives an attack it enters the five *zang.* When it enters the six *fu,* the body becomes warm or hot, and you can't remain lying down quietly because the perversion is on the *biao,* in a movement towards the exterior. If there is some kind of rising to the top, there is dyspnoea - problems with breathing. When it enters the five *zang,* there is dilation, congestion and swelling, because it is a movement towards the interior, *li.* There are blockages and obstructions, and when it descends towards the lower part of the trunk it gives diarrhoea with undigested food. If it lasts a long time then there are different kinds of flowing out such as dysentery. That is a complete disturbance in the ways of the clear and unclear inside the body.

The Emperor said:

When the Spleen is ill the four limbs are out of use, why is this?

And Qi Bo replied:

The four limbs receive the Breaths of the Stomach

The ideogram for receive is *lin ,* the same ideogram which is the active part of the distribution and reception of something and this idea of receiving something is exactly the same as the idea of receiving grains from granaries to nourish the people. The four limbs receive Breaths from the Stomach in the same way that a part of the Empire receives a public distribution of grains.

But the Breaths of the Stomach cannot reach the meridians without the support of the Spleen which is absolutely necessary to it.

We see that the Stomach is *yang,* in the image of the Breaths of Heaven, but after the *yang* movement of the Stomach we need the movement and distribution of the Spleen in order that the Breaths of the

Stomach can go deep in to the body and out to the four limbs or to the *zang* and *fu*. The Breaths of the Stomach can descend by their own movement and can be transmitted to the Intestines and so on, but it's necessary that the Spleen intervenes and that there is interplay between the Spleen and Stomach.

Then there can be distribution and reception.....

....which is the same ideogram, *lin*. It means distribution from a Centre, from the Stomach and Spleen, and reception by the four limbs.

津液
脉

When the Spleen is ill the Stomach is unable to make the jin ye circulate. The four limbs no longer receive the Breaths from the liquids and cereals. The Breaths decrease day by day and the pathways of the mai no longer function. The muscles and the bones and the flesh are all without breath to give them life. This is why they are out of use.

Why is this important for the four limbs? Because the four limbs are the place for the twelve meridians and the activity of *yang* Breaths, and through and by the *yang* Breaths all the exterior activity of the body is possible. You know that the important five Element points are located from the extremities to the first articulation so it is important that this region is well irrigated and well maintained in order to be able to support needling.

If a man doesn't eat and no longer has enough Breaths of the Stomach, or if his Spleen is injured and cannot distribute influx and nutrition to muscles, bones and flesh, out to the extremities of the four limbs, then there is no activity in this man. Also it will be quite impossible to needle him, particularly at the extremities of the limbs because there is no circulation and no passage through the *mai*.

Then the Emperor takes up another question:

The Spleen doesn't govern a season, can you explain this to me?

Qi Bo replies:

94

The Spleen is the Earth, tu, it governs the central region, and continually through the four seasons it allows the development of the four zang.

This is quite important. It's not only through the Breaths of the Stomach that the four or five *zang* can remain alive and function. The Spleen masters the four seasons and all these qualities of Breaths which form time and moments, and by virtue of this Spleen can give force to the four other *zang*. The Spleen governs eighteen days in each season or rather Spleen is entrusted with eighteen days in each season, it does not command one single season. The Spleen ensures a good passage from one quality of Breaths to another quality of Breaths, from one season to another and one *zang* to another. By itself, Spleen has no ability to master one season, its particular virtue is to master the time of passages and transmissions. For this reason the Spleen masters eighteen days in each season, and these days are between two seasons. There is no contradiction with the fact that in other texts in the Nei Jing or in other presentations Spleen masters the so-called long Summer, because long Summer - the end or the prolongation of the Summer - is the time in the year during which *yang* seasons become *yin* seasons, and this is essentially a time for passage. It's a time and a space where the movement of *yin* and *yang* is reversed. At the beginning of Autumn the Breaths of Heaven rise up and leave Earth and the Breaths of Earth concentrate and descend: it's the beginning of the separation of Heaven and Earth. And you can find the opposite movement in Springtime. In both cases the Earth Element, Spleen and Stomach, masters this time of change, transformation, permutation and passage.

The Earth Element contains all the possibility for exchange that we can see between Heaven and Earth. For this reason, inside the quality and virtue of the Earth Element we have ascending and descending movement, we have the occupation of the head as well as the foot. This Earth Element is omnipresent in the seasons, in each moment of time where one quality of Breaths has to pass to another quality of Breaths , and in all parts of space where transformations, permutations and passages have to take place. This is the reason why Spleen and Stomach are joined in a very important interplay, because in the body they are the exact image of the interplay of Heaven and Earth; ascending and descending, diffusing and concentrating, and all the separations between clear and unclear.

You may see with other quotations from the Nei Jing how Spleen and Stomach are necessary for the renewal of the *zang* and *fu, yin* and *yang,* meridians, Spirits, Essences, Blood and Breaths. And for this reason if Earth or Spleen is in the central position it means that it has no one special place, but all places which are pivots between two qualities of Breaths.

At the end of the chapter the Emperor asks:

津液

The Spleen and Stomach are connected by the tissues and membranes that attach them together. It is through this that there can be the circulation of jin ye.

It's necessary that this close connection between Spleen and Stomach is manifest in the membranes that attach them together. That is the density of relationships in Earth, that they are so closely related that there is actually a physical connection, and it gives them mastery over all the circulations which take place through these tissues or membranes. The Emperor asks if the circulation of bodily liquids is actually passed by this kind of tissue or membrane into all parts of the body and especially into the trunk and between the viscera. Qi Bo replies:

脈
絡

The tai yin of the foot is the third yin, its mai passes through the Stomach and takes a dependent relationship with the Spleen, and a luo connecting relation with the throat. And so it is that the tai yin is that which makes the Breaths circulate to the three yin and the yang ming is the biao, the movement to the exterior, the sea of the five zang and six fu. It's also that which makes the Breaths circulate to the three yang.

This is a recollection of what we said before about the responsibility of the Stomach and Spleen for the three *yang* meridians and the three *yin* meridians, or the twelve meridians, and the Breaths of the Stomach being the Sea of the five *zang* and the six *fu* and for all meridians and Breaths of meridians. In that interplay between Stomach and Spleen,

Spleen has the responsibility for circulation and the sensation of circulation and function of *yin* meridians, and the Stomach the same for the *yang* meridians.

 The zang and the fu each of them, receive Breaths through the yang ming, so it is the Stomach that makes the jin ye circulate.

We just saw that for the circulation of bodily liquids Stomach needs the help of the Spleen in order to have the *yin* movement and the *yang* movement acting together to irrigate and water all the body.

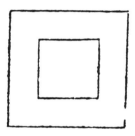

扶突天突旁五寸禾髎水髎旁五分迎香禾髎

上二寸大腸經穴 是分明

胃者水穀氣血之海也○

大一尺五寸徑五寸長二尺

六寸橫屈受水穀應該三斗

五升其中之穀常留二斗水

一斗五升而滿○是經多氣

多血○難經曰胃重二觔十四兩

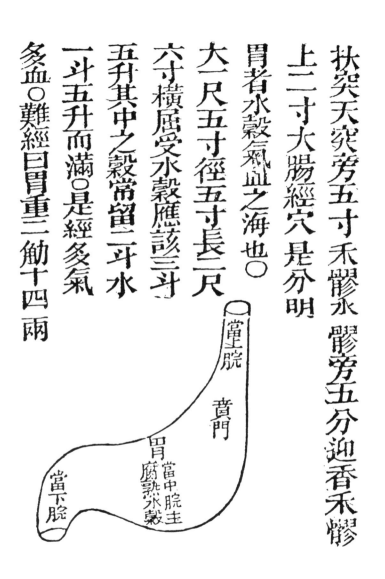

The Stomach from the Ling Shu Su Wen Jie Yao

THE STOMACH

Ling Shu Chapter 30

津液脉 *The six Breaths of the human body are Essences, Breaths, jin, ye, Blood and mai.*

Elisabeth Rochat: Breaths can be seen as part of the 'six Breaths' because Breaths can be understood at many levels. At the most general level they are a way by which life takes place and remains, but you can also take Breaths, *qi,* at another level, and at this general level, *qi* is the general sign of animation. In this case, besides animation, you have Essences, nutrition, the liquid aspect, the circulating aspect, and so on. So for this reason we can call Breaths all that makes life,, and we can divide these breaths into several aspects of which Breaths, *qi,* represents only one aspect of animation.

The six Breaths are Essences, Breaths, *jin, ye,* Blood and *mai.* Each of these six Breaths has its particular region of mastery, and they all have their relative positions which have different roles in the good or bad state of the organism.

So it is that the five cereals and the Stomach are the big Sea for all of this.

This is a way of saying that all that makes life in a person has its seed, its origin, its reserve in the Stomach and through the Stomach, not only the meridians, *zang fu,* and so on, but also these six Breaths.

This expression to be a Sea is very clear in Ling Shu Chapter 33:

氣街
三里

膻中

衝脉

The Stomach is the Sea of liquids and cereals. Its point of action at a distance is above at the road of Breaths (qi jie, Stomach 30) and below at san li (Stomach 36).

The important point is that it is one of the four Seas, Brain (Sea of Marrow), *tan zhong* (Sea of Breaths), Stomach (Sea of Liquids and Cereals), and *chong mai* (Sea of Twelve Meridians or Sea of Blood). This is very interesting because *chong mai* and Stomach have two very close connections. In Ling Shu Chapter 33, *chong mai* is one time called the Sea of Twelve Meridians, and another time called the Sea of Blood, and in fact *chong mai* is the Sea of a lot of things! It is the Sea of the *zang* and *fu,* and the Stomach also is called the Sea of the five *zang* and six *fu.* You'll remember that the pathway of *chong mai* passes through the region of Stomach 30, rises up along the abdomen and doubles along the pathway of the Stomach meridian and the Kidney meridian. But the special function of *chong mai* is to be the Root of Anterior and Posterior Heaven, and of the Kidneys' and Stomach's functions.

You can see that the Stomach is the only viscera in this series of Four Seas, and it is really a *fu,* because it receives exterior food and begins to engage the process of transformation, digestion, assimilation and the extraction of Essences.

For this reason we have other chapters, like Ling Shu Chapter 60, which say:

The Breaths that man receives are the cereals.....

It's very clear - if you want to have Breaths you need some basis for the assimilation and transformation of food.

....and the place where the cereals pour out is the Stomach. The Stomach is the Sea of Breaths and Blood which come from liquids and cereals. The Breaths from the clouds which come from the seas are everywhere under Heaven.

We can see in that an explanation of the meaning of 'Sea'. It's a place for exchange between Heaven and Earth because from the sea evaporation can take place and the Breaths of Earth rise up to Heaven and form clouds, and afterwards the clouds will give rain, rain descends to the Earth and forms rivers and rivers return to the sea. Influx coming from the sea fulfils Heaven and Earth.

Claude Larre: Wind is also necessary because if it was just an exchange between sea and Heaven, ascending and descending, there would be no fertilization on Earth as such. And the sea? I would refer you to Lao Zi when they talk of the one hundred rivers which gently flow towards the sea. They use it in a political manner to say that tributary states have to report to them. Or they would say that in an analogical manner all the currents they are describing in the human body finally have to return to one of the Four Seas.

Elisabeth Rochat: In Ling Shu Chapter 60 it is interesting to see that the Stomach is named Sea of Breaths and Blood, of all vitality and all that circulates in the meridians. The end of this quotation is:

The Breaths and Blood which come out of the Stomach, these are the ditches.

 The meaning of the word *sui,* ditches or trenches, is that a meridian is a circulation of Blood, of Breaths, and various qualities of Breaths such as nutritive and defensive. It's exactly the same as in a large town now, we have circulation by cables for electricity, phones, gas, water, heating and so on, and all these kinds of cables or threads are in a sort of ditch.

Claude Larre: Ditches are casements for putting in a series of different influxes. They cut the crust of the Earth, dig a sizeable place and make a casement, through which everything goes. So it's less a ditch as such, than the ditch and the work and the final result with everything going more or less in the same direction.

Elisabeth Rochat: There is a Chinese expression, ditches of meridians, which has the meaning of designating all kinds of circulation which take place through meridians, Breaths, Blood, nutrition, defence, and these ditches, these channels, are the great network of relations of the five *zang* and six *fu*. Or you can take the same sentence in the singular not the plural, this ditch is the great connecting network, the great *luo* for the five *zang* and six *fu*. It's impossible to decide with only the Chinese text whether we should use the singular or the plural form. We will see this later in Su Wen Chapter 18 when we discuss the great *luo* of the Stomach.

But now for some more quotations

 The Stomach is the great granary, da cang, the great storehouse. The five orifices of the Stomach are the great and small doors of villages and hamlets.

102

This is a very strange formulation. The meaning is that the Stomach has five orifices which are under its responsibility - the pharynx, the cardia, the pyloric sphincter, the ileo-cecal valve and the anus. This is important because we see from this that the mastership of the Stomach extends from the pharynx, the first entry point of food, to the anus, the exit point of food, passing through all articulations and passages between oesophagus and Stomach, between Stomach and Small Intestine, and between Small Intestine and Large Intestine, and finally between exterior and interior, and interior and exterior. As a result we have two points with a particular action for the Small and Large Intestine, Stomach 37 and 39.

Peter Firebrace: Stomach 37 and 39 are sometimes called Sea of Blood along with Bladder 11.

衝脉 *Elisabeth Rochat:*   We can find something about that in Ling Shu Chapter 33, the chapter on the Four Seas. If you remember, *chong mai* is called the Sea of Blood in this chapter, and the points for particular action on the Sea of Blood are Bladder 11 and Stomach 37 and 39. That might be the link in the text - but in this chapter it is in particular relationship with *chong mai,* it's not directly linked with Stomach, although we saw that Stomach and *chong mai* have a very strong relationship and perhaps *chong mai* is like an ancestor or a producer of what in a perfectly formed man, should be the function of the Stomach: *chong mai* is like a prefiguration of that.

In some texts, *yang ming,* the Stomach meridian, appears like a chief, important for headmastering all the meridians, or all the *yang* meridians.

Su Wen Chapter 34

Yang ming is the mai of the Stomach,
and Stomach is the Sea of the six fu

Su Wen Chapter 44

宗筋 *Yang ming is the Sea of the five zang and six fu, it masters and waters the Ancestral Muscle, zong jin. Ancestral Muscle masters the bones that make a chain and it ensures the subtle mechanisms of all articulations and joints. It is a place of reunion and connection for all muscular forces in the body, and the commanding place for the muscles.*

This is especially expressed in the attachment of all the muscles and bones which are so visible along the back in the vertebral column. The text continues:

Yang ming is the Sea of the five zang and six fu, and this yang ming masters and waters the Ancestral Muscle. Chong mai is the Sea of Meridians and it masters the irrigation and humidification of great and small valleys.

氣街 *Chong mai* makes a junction with *yang ming* in the region of the Ancestral Muscle. *Yin* and *yang* are gathered together and this gathering occurs in the region of *qi jie,* Street of Breaths, Stomach 30. But also this is the name given to a very important region which gives a good circulation of Breaths, and *yang ming* is the headmaster of this region.

絡 帶脈 All these regions and all these functions have a relationship of 督脈 dependence with *dai mai* and a relationship of *luo* (connection) with *du mai,* and for this reason, if *yang ming* is empty then the Ancestral Muscle is loosened, and *dai mai* can no longer ensure good directing

104

power. Consequently, the inferior members become impotent with flaccidity and can no longer be used. The importance of this is that the power of *yang ming* is necessary for all meridians and also for the extraordinary meridians, *chong mai, dai mai,* and *du mai.* It is also important for the whole movement of the body because *yang ming* masters and irrigates the *zong jin,* and this Ancestral Muscle is exactly like a point of gathering and mastering for all that is muscular in the body. It's necessary to have *yang ming,* to have movement, to have good articulation, to have good links between flesh and muscle and so on. I think this is the important point, that not only the twelve meridians but also the extraordinary meridians need *yang ming.*

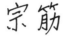

Ancestral Muscle, *zong jin.*

Elisabeth Rochat: *Zong jin* is very interesting: it's the power inside the muscle, the connection between flesh and bones and the power for movement. It's not a muscle in the meaning of a muscular mass, it's the muscular power.

Claude Larre: It's the same question as Blood and animation. There is no real Blood without animation, and no real muscle without this *zong jin.*

Elisabeth Rochat: It's called ancestral, but what's the real meaning of an ancestor? An ancestor or the grandfather in a family is able to gather all the members together for special circumstances, for discussions or birthdays or special ceremonies. And sometimes this grandfather has some ideas on the state of the family or the right conduct of affairs and he can give direction. He has a kind of mastership of the family and he makes the spirit of the family. He forms the link between all members of the family because he's also the origin, all the sons come from him, so he is the one who gathers them together and commands or directs them, and also conducts worship to the family ancestors. This is the meaning of this ideogram *zong*. And *zong jin* is the Ancestral Muscle, but it's not exactly an accurate translation because muscle is not muscle and ancestor is not ancestor in this particular context. *Zong jin* is a very archaic mechanism of the body from which all expression of muscular power occurs in the organism. The best example of this muscular power is the penis with the phenomenon of erection, but it also occurs in every part of the body where a link, or tie between bones and flesh exists, or where there is articulation and movement.

宗脉
宗氣

Also, at the level of the brain, the Sea of Marrow, or more precisely in the area of the eyes and the ears, we have *zong mai*, and this place has for the *mai* this same effect of commanding and gathering; and in *tan zhong*, the Sea of Breaths, we have *zong qi*, ancestral Breaths and in this Sea of Breaths there is the power of gathering and commanding all the Breaths of the body; and of course *zong jin* has a relationship with *chong mai* and Stomach, the other two Seas.

Su Wen Chapter 18

Elisabeth Rochat: This chapter deals with the change and transformation of *yin yang* and the four seasons which have very important repercussions on the human body and particularly on the beating of the mai, the pulse.

Because of these repercussions, Chinese medicine differentiates four different sorts of pulses according to the four seasons. But beyond that, these four pulses, differentiated according to the four *zang* and the four seasons, are rooted in the Breaths of the Stomach.

脉

The aspect that my pulse presents always has to be even and very supple, well harmonized and well-tempered. If in each aspect presented by the *mai*, the Breaths of the Stomach are too weak, it's a sign of disease, and if there are no longer any Breaths of Stomach it is a sign of

106

death. For the *mai,* the Breaths of the Stomach are like a root.

The great *luo* of the Stomach, *xu li*

It is in this context that the presentation of the great *luo* of the Stomach appears. The first thing must be to ask what exactly is the meaning of *luo?* It's like a network, a connection, or a special relationship between two things or two functions which are not the same but which have exactly the same quality of Breaths, and which can be complementary. For example, this *luo* connection is specific to the relationship between a meridian and the viscera with which the meridian is in a couple, for instance, the Spleen meridian has a *luo* connection with the Stomach, and the Stomach meridian a *luo* connection with the Spleen.

Among the *luo* there are fifteen great *luo*. These great *luo* stem from the meridians which are the great directional pattern of circulation of Breaths and the guarantee of the good quality of each type of Breath, *tai, shao* or *jue yin* and *tai, shao* or *yang ming*. The Great *luo* are special connections between two meridians which are in interplay in a *biao li* relationship because they are the twofold aspect of one Element, for example Stomach and Spleen.

A *luo* is not only these things but also the function of connecting this quality of Breaths of meridians with a special part of the body. The *luo* of the Bladder is very short but the *luo* of the Heart Master, for example, is very long and very important. From the point *nei guan* it ensures relationship with the Triple Heater meridian, and also the relationship through the communication with the Heart, with all the internal viscera.

We can also see the ideogram *luo* in all circulations which are not meridian circulations. There are infinite branches or ramifications right up to the most superficial aspects of the body.

107

心包絡

督脉
任脉
大包

We also saw this ideogram *luo* when we studied the Heart as Master, *xin bao luo,* with the function of enveloping and protecting the Heart and ensuring connections and communications of the Spirit of the Heart with all the other aspects of the organism, in particular the *zang* .

The Stomach has a normal great *luo,* one of the fifteen great *luo* explained in Ling Shu Chapter 10. Of the fifteen, twelve are related to the twelve meridians, one to *du mai,* one to *ren mai,* and the fifteenth is the great *luo* of the Spleen, *da bao,* which means great envelope. The ideogram *bao* is the same as in *xin bao luo* - sometimes the radical changes but it is this same idea of an envelope. *Da bao* starts on the sides of the body, it anchors the two sides of the body and spreads out in the direction of the ribs and the thorax. It is that which gathers together and envelopes, and which has the possibility of bringing together everything which is a network or communication, *luo,* and which is therefore able to link in with the internal *zang* through its connecting power. It's a kind of enveloping matrix which is at the level of the thorax and which develops from the exterior and penetrates into the interior. This is very interesting because we will see a completely different movement with *xu li,* the great *luo* of the Stomach.

虚里

The text of Su Wen Chapter 18 says:

絡
虚里
脉

The great luo of the Stomach, its name is xu li. It crosses through the diaphragm and takes a connecting relationship with the Lung. It comes out under the left breast. Its movement beats under the clothes. It is the Ancestral Breaths of the mai.

大包

You can see that that great *luo* of the Stomach, in contrast to the great *luo* of the Spleen, *da bao,* is central in its position. It is not anchored on both sides but just springs out from the Middle Heater and passes through the middle of the diaphragm: the movement of very refined Breaths and Essences of the Middle Heater rising up, ascending to the Upper Heater. The movement is the contrary to the great *luo* of the Spleen which is rather like an external envelope penetrating to the intimate life, while this great *luo* of the Stomach begins in the more intimate depths, moving through the diaphragm coming to the level of

膻中 the Sea of Breaths, *tan zhong,* and coming out under the left breast. So it leaves the central position and moves to the left. Why to the left? Simply because it's the place of the Heart. This *luo* is like the source of Ancestral Breaths, and the Ancestral Breaths activate the Breaths and give the beating movement to the Heart: it is the beating of the Heart which is this beating under the clothes. Through the beating of the Heart and the functioning of the Lung all Breaths are distributed through the circuit of the twelve meridians.

宗氣 We saw previously the special relationship of the Stomach thanks to the great *luo, xu li,* with the Sea of Breaths and *zong qi,* the Ancestral Breaths, which are able to activate rhythmic circulation in the form of the circulation of the meridians, beating of the Heart and respiration. There is also a connection between the Middle and Upper Heaters, just as before there was a connection between the Middle and Lower Heaters with the Ancestral Muscle.

虛里
建里 Before we go any further, let's take a look at the ideograms *xu li,* because they are so important. *Xu* is not an envelope, it is a void. I prefer this term void to empty. And *li* is an intimate structuration - though intimate structuration is not the exact translation. You will remember the name of the point *ren mai* 11, *jian li.* This is the same *li* ideogram, and *jian* has the meaning of to firmly establish something. Its location is just before the special point for the Stomach, *ren mai* 12, and this is perhaps the connection.

氣
里 The Stomach is the great Sea for the five *zang* and the six *fu,* the great Sea for Blood and *qi,* the great Sea for cereals and liquids etc, so it is the place for the establishment of all renewal of the intimate structure of life. I think this is the meaning of the *li* ideogram, the construction of a very deep and intimate living relationship which is very well organized.

Claude Larre: It's difficult to isolate the meaning of *li* from *xu* or from *jian* because if you are describing an effect, this effect is in the median and there is no way to talk of the median except by talking of what makes the median - that is the two characters together.The difficulty is

里
建
虚

that we want two things at the same time, we want to understand what *li* is and we want to understand why they use this character. Because if they use this character it's because it's used in the median where life is establishing itself. So one may ask what do you really want? Do you want to know what *li* is or do you want to know what *li* is in that particular configuration? And then it is necessary to come back to *jian* or *xu,* because there is no meaning without them.

宗氣

Elisabeth Rochat: Life, Breaths, assimilation, animation and distribution of influences can only appear through void, or voids, and perhaps this void is an allusion to the Heart? It's from the Stomach and the Middle Heater, and through the Sea of Breaths of the Upper Heater that these Breaths called Ancestral Breaths, *zong qi,* take form and allow the beating of the Heart, all of which is a manifestation that this man is alive and not dead. But the structuration, *li,* is coming from the Stomach. We can also say that the Centre or the central region has to be a void, in exactly the same manner as the wheel needs a void Centre in order to function.

Claude Larre: I would like to relate this to the Mawangdui Banner. We've recently been preparing a commentary on the banner based around the idea that if you cut the banner from top to bottom, there is an axis, and at this axis either it is revolving or it is void. So when Elisabeth is making a comparison between the necessity of the void in the Heart and the necessity of *xu li* which is connected with the Stomach, she is just saying the same thing. Whenever life has to be expressed with fullness in relation to two different points of view, one has to be this central sovereign quality of the whole authority of the Heart. In these two cases the configuration of the organization must be the same. If there is no void there is no circulation, if there is no circulation there is no life. In the banner it is the same because if the banner relates to the prayer of the people, it can't be done except through the void, because how can you circulate prayers, or how can you really pass from this world to the other world, or how could you be accepted there if there is not a place for this movement? So the representation of

110

the banner has the same quality of central void as Lao Zi with the wheel.

Elisabeth Rochat: This void is also the only way to have a Centre for distribution, and an expression like "the crossroads of the four voids" appears in some classical philosophical texts. The idea is that only a void allows distribution in the four directions for communication. In the case of the Stomach it is at the level of the Sea of liquids and cereals, Blood and Breaths, twelve meridians, *zang* and *fu,* for the renewal of life.

Now, I just want to justify the reason why I said previously that perhaps the void was alluding to the Heart. If you look at the Kidney meridian points 23, 24 and 25, in the names of 23 and 25 you have *shen,* spirits, which are connected with the Heart, and the name of Kidney 24 is *ling xu. Ling* is spiritual influx and *xu* is the same as before, the void. Just add the radical of Earth and the meaning is like a place for a city, but the place of this city or void is obviously the Heart, because we are in the place of the Heart and its function, and this point is just between two points with the name *shen,* spirits.

You can see that Breaths of the organism in the five *zang* need Breaths from the Stomach, and these Breaths of each of the five *zang* are gathered in the Sea of Breaths in the middle of the chest, and there is a special, direct relationship between Stomach and this Sea of Breaths thanks to the great *luo* of the Stomach, *xu li.* For this reason *zong qi,* Ancestral Breaths, are really the summation of all kinds of Breaths able to manage life in the organism, and when the text adds:

it is the Ancestral Breaths of the mai

the meaning is that the Ancestral Breaths are like a starting point of the circulation through the meridians, and it's also the Ancestral Breaths of the pulses. You know that the ideogram *mai* has this two-fold meaning, so when you take the pulses, you have to consider the state of the Breaths of the Stomach, and how they present in the particular pulse of each *zang* and *fu.* This is the meaning in Su Wen Chapter 18.

111

You can see this situation of the Ancestral Breaths more clearly with the participation of the Stomach in the middle of the chest, and through the beating of the Heart. This is the sign of life. Chapter 18 says:

中積

When it overflows in fullness, whether there is panting, or whether it is frequent and interrupted, the illness is at the Centre, zhong.When it is knotted and transversal, there are accumulations, ji.

In this case transversal is the idea of going astray, or not in a good way.

絶
宗氣

If it is interrupted, jue, and no longer arrives, it is death. Under the breast its movement is echoed in the clothes: it is the Ancestral Breaths, zong qi, that flow out.

If the Ancestral Breaths are the summation of the Essences and Breaths that are necessary to live, it's evident that these kinds of Breaths must remain in circulation in the organism and never flow out. If they flow out there is a loss of vitality, and there's no more circulation in the *mai.* You can feel that on the pulses, and you can feel that simply through the beating of the Heart. The pulses are also the expression of the movement of the Heart, and the Heart masters the *mai,* with this two-fold meaning of network of animation and circulation of Breaths and Blood and pulses.

脉

If you want an explanation of the pathological aspect of Ancestral Breaths we can say that when they overflow in fullness there is a very strong beating of the Heart. Sometimes we can have bad respiration and this is a sign that some perverse activity is taking place in the Ancestral Breaths and *xu li.* This word "panting" means bad respiration, but perhaps this kind of very strong beating of the Heart is also indicated in this particular case. When it's frequent, it's too fast, and it's a great and perverse intensity.

虚里

Intermittent means that sometimes there is an interruption, it's not an indefinite interruption, but it's a great irregularity in respiration, the beating of the pulses and the circulation of Blood and Breaths through the Heart. These illnesses are in the Centre. What is the meaning of this

膻中 Centre? Perhaps it is the Stomach? Perhaps it is the Centre of the chest, *tan zhong?* Perhaps it is the Heart? I think that the meaning of the Centre in this case is not well defined, but maybe it is just the intimate Centre of vitality, with a connection with the Stomach and the Ancestral Breaths, through Lung and Heart.

中 *Claude Larre:* It comes down to the same question we were talking about before, the internal and external not being on the same level. It is impossible to represent with actual location, the inner, but what is true of inner is also somewhat true of *zhong*. But there is a difference in whether this inner is in relation to something which is not itself in space and which is not said to be concentrated somewhere. When you say *zhong,* middle, it's necessarily inner, but it's more than inner, it's the space from where everything starts, from where directions are given, and it's a place where all my special powers are gathered under my ancestors' guidance, under Heaven's mandate and the gathering of all the Spirits. And the most special and extraordinary things that may come to me come to the Centre, the *zhong*.

Zong qi and the six Breaths

宗氣 *Question:* I have a question from earlier which is not clear. Would you compare or contrast *zong qi* with the six Breaths?

Elisabeth Rochat: Zong qi, Ancestral Breaths, are a mechanism of all the Breaths which are renewed in and through the organism. You can call them Breaths of Posterior Heaven.

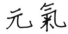 *Claude Larre:* Elisabeth is insisting on Posterior Heaven because there are other breaths, the *yuan qi* which are of Anterior Heaven. So if *zong qi* is ascribed to Posterior Heaven it's just because the true origin of life

113

is the origin of the universe, which is necessarily called Anterior Heaven. It means that before anything can exist in me or elsewhere it is necessary to prepare this distinction between Heaven and Earth in the chaos.

元氣

宗氣

If we say "before I myself existed" it is not the same. You can say that for myself there is a non-existing state, *yuan qi*, which is preserved in me after I am born. It is the same with embryology, which is still having an effect on my life after I am an adult. Now, after my birth, I am still governed by *yuan qi*, but this *yuan qi* in being contrasted with other *qi*, is contrasted first with *zong qi*. Then *zong qi* is understood to be the connective device to preserve the ancestral mind in myself and to make myself me, because *yuan qi* does not aim to conserve or preserve the characteristics of my personality. *Yuan qi* is the origin of my life, while *zong qi* is the specific origin my life and this specification proceeds from the fact that I am a man, that I am a man of this time, from that lineage, and that I am this particular individual. All that comes under the rubric of *zong qi*. There is then no conflict between *yuan qi* and *zong qi*, but the point of view is not the same. And if the point of view is not the same you have a different character for it. But just because you have two different Chinese characters you are not supposed to make such a contrast that you think that they are opposite! They are contrasted but they are the same, it's the same reality, but it's not seen from the same angle.

Elisabeth Rochat: It is because *zong qi* is related to Posterior Heaven that the link between Stomach and *zong qi* is so strong, because the Stomach and Spleen are the root and trunk for posterior Heaven in the body.

Claude Larre: But Tim was asking about the relationship between *zong qi* and the six Breaths.

津液 *Elisabeth Rochat:* The six Breaths are Essences, Breaths, *jin, ye,*

114

脈
津液

Blood and *mai*. We can have three couples or three dual expressions: Essences/Breaths, *jin ye*, Blood/*mai*. *Mai* being the storehouse for Blood. You see that these six Breaths, or forms of life are everywhere. There are Essences everywhere in the body, Essences from Anterior Heaven and Posterior Heaven, and the patterns and mechanisms for the renewal of Breaths are all a kind of animation, an ascending and diffusing movement from the Centre to the periphery, bringing power, strength and warmth. *Jin ye* are exactly the same mechanism between the renewal of the matter of life and animation, but at the level of the bodily liquids, giving animation, circulation, nutrition, irrigation and watering in a diffusing movement. Blood and *mai* are the last couple. For this animation by the *mai* and for this red liquid full of life and the Spirit of the Heart, you need the work of the Spleen and Stomach. You know that through the richest and finest juices coming from the Spleen, rising up to the Lung and being offered to the Heart, Blood can be renewed. Why is there this dividing of the vitality of the body into six? Because six is the number for exchange and for maintenance in a very well defined space.

氣

Claude Larre: The Chinese either take *qi* as the big mass of everything which we are concerned with for life, or they take it under the Heaven/Earth/ Man relationship, and this would necessarily come under the number six. Six is for relations. When you take one for one the relationship is not seen. It doesn't mean that there is no relationship but it is not explicit. The big problem in talking about acupuncture in English or French is whether we are ready to look at the same thing under different aspects or not. If we are ready we need a guide, and the guide will be that five is five and six is six, and five is not six and six is not five, except in cases where five is six and six is five! And what seems to be ridiculous is just that. We are ridiculous, it's not what I say that is ridiculous. We are ridiculous because we are asking Chinese people to force their minds and practice into our own model.

Elisabeth Rochat:

When it is knotted and transversal there are accumulations

脉

A knot is a very irregular frequency. This kind of accumulation can be very varied. We can have accumulations in the area of the Heart or in the abdomen, or in the Stomach or the region of the diaphragm. We can have local *mai* with or without strength. For example, if we have a kind of sensation of pulsing or beating, irregular but with great strength, there is a blockage in the circulation. There are sometimes clottings, with the blockage taking a shape, because there is this perverse fullness. If the aspect is knotted and very weak it may be after a long illness with a great loss of liquids or Blood. Or if there is a powerful and strong emotion such as fear and the Spirits disperse and are unable to gather again, you will have the impression of weakness and irregularity, because of the connection of the pulses and *mai* with the Heart, and through the Heart to the Spirits of the Heart. Sometimes when the Breaths of the Heart are damaged by one cause or another this can effect the proper movement through the *zong qi* and the activity of *xu li,* and there is an accumulation. Then there is no good activity from the Stomach and no good distribution to the *zang* and *fu* and to the Breaths and so on to renew Essences and vitality.

宗氣
虛里

Under the breast its movement is echoed in the clothes.

膻中

When you can feel the beating of the Heart too much, it's a sign that the Ancestral Breaths are flowing out and no longer keeping within the Sea of Breaths, *tan zhong.* They are in a state of over-excitement, an over speeding up, and you know what happens with a horse or a machine in this state!

I think that this chapter is clear now; the connection of the Stomach and *xu li* with the Lung, Ancestral Breaths, respiration and distribution of influx through the Sea of Breaths, the beating of the Heart, and, of course, life and death.

116

The five zang receive the Breaths distributed from the Stomach. The Stomach is the root of the five zang.

This is an important point, the Breaths of the five *zang* cannot arrive by themselves at the *tai yin* of the hand. The meaning is that to arrive at the *tai yin* of the hand, where they can be felt on the radial pulse, they need the effect produced by the Breaths of the Stomach. Another way to say exactly the same thing is that it happens through *xu li* and the Breaths of the Stomach with its special ascending movement. The Breaths of the Stomach release the most subtle Essences for the renewal of life for the five *zang* and six *fu*, through meridians and through *zong qi*. It is through this that all the variety of Breaths, in particular of the five *zang*, can be felt on the radial pulse through the *tai yin* of the hand. The pulse is also the way by which you can see the equilibrium between *yin* and *yang* in the shape of Blood and Breaths, and the strength of circulation in the quality and quantity of this red liquid.

虚里
宗氣

Ling Shu Chapter 56

Another thing is that from the Stomach not only *zong qi* but also nutritive and defensive Breaths are renewed. This is very clearly said in Ling Shu Chapter 56:

The Stomach is the Sea of the five zang and six fu, liquids and cereals all enter the Stomach. The five zang and six fu all receive the Breaths of the Stomach. The five Tastes each go to the place that pleases them. The cereals of which the taste is acid go by preference to the Liver, they are attracted by the Liver. Those of the bitter taste go to the Heart, Those of sweet to the Spleen, those of acrid to the Lung, and those of salty to the Kidneys. The Breaths of the cereals and the jin ye that come from them circulate. The ying wei, the nutritive and defensive, or nutrition and

津液
營衛

defence, circulate freely everywhere. Then through transformation there are the residues and wastes which are directed as they must, below.

The important point is that the Stomach is really the turning point for the releasing of Breaths in the form of Ancestral Breaths, for the renewal of the *zang* in the form of the five Tastes, the bodily liquids, and defensive and nutritive Breaths, and finally, also in the form of the separation of the wastes and disposal.

Ling Shu Chapter 28

宗脉

宗筋
宗氣

In Ling Shu Chapter 28 it is said that the eye and the ear are special places for the accumulation of the Ancestral *mai, zong mai*. It follows that when there is a great emptiness in the middle of the Stomach, then the *zong mai* are empty, and being empty, all flows downwards and the *mai* become like a spring that dries up. For this reason we have a kind of buzzing in the ear. We now have the final relationship with the *zong* activity in the body. We saw the relationship of the Stomach with the Ancestral Muscle, *zong jin,* with the Ancestral Breaths, *zong qi,* and now we have a text pointing out the relationship of the Stomach with the Ancestral *mai, zong mai*. We have covered the middle of the chest, the upper part of the abdomen, and now we are in this part of the head, with the brain involved too. Here it is not only an external ear, but an internal ear, and it's the same for the eyes. So why do the *zong mai* have a special relationship with this part of the body, not only with the Heart and the Sea of Breaths, but also with the eye and the ear, and with the finest Essences of the brain. The *mai* are an expression of radiance, the radiance which is the radiance of the Spirits through the Essences by the Heart or by the brain. It's the power of the Stomach shown in the rising up of the finest Breaths , and for this reason there is the pathway of the Stomach meridian on the head and connected with the orifices (see Ling Shu Chapter 62). This also shows why the pulse of the Stomach is so important, because it governs all this movement over the head.

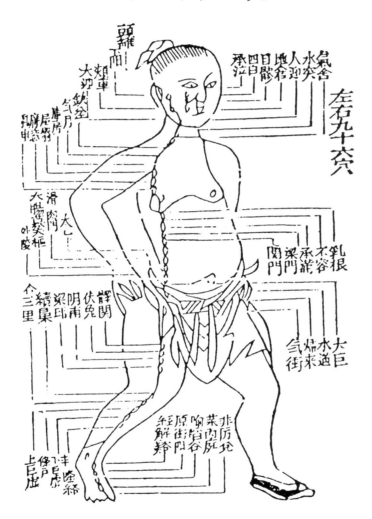

The *zu yang ming* Stomach meridian from the Ling Shu Su Wen Jie Yao

119

Functions of the Spleen and Stomach

Elisabeth Rochat: We've seen that the Spleen and Stomach are essential in all physiological functions of man, and therefore that the Spleen and Stomach will often have a very essential role in physiology, pathology and symptomatology. A quotation from a very famous twelfth century book, the Treatise on the Spleen and Stomach says:

That which offers the yin and the Essences is Spleen and Stomach, and this is in harmonious conjunction with their Breaths. The Breaths from the cereals rise up and its circulation follows the movement of Spring and Summer, the movement where yang is rising for life. And it is in this way that man reaches longevity. And on the contrary if there is disharmony between Spleen and Stomach there will be the loss or inability to grasp the Essences so that all the thesaurizations will be impoverished, and this will give a premature death.

運化 We've seen that the two ideograms which summed up the characteristics of Spleen were *yun hua,* transportation or distribution, and transformation. Therefore they are concerned with all the progression of digestion and assimilation. But this word transformation is not only used for digestion and assimilation and the digestive process, but also for all kinds of adaptations, when you have a change in your life, for example, or the adaptation to a new kind of food. It's the idea of making use of all the elements that are at your disposal.

化 *Claude Larre:* The highest meaning of *hua* is seen in the Lie Zi Chapter 1, where *hua* is the creative transforming power.

Elisabeth Rochat: This function of transporting and transforming is seen in two aspects. The first aspect is the specific action of the Spleen,

精微

helped by the Stomach, on the *jing wei,* the subtle Essences, and this is the same for the distribution of the five Tastes through the body to each of the *zang*.

Another aspect of this function of transforming and transporting is on the specific action on the liquids and dampness or humidity in the body. Contemporary Chinese books talk about its action on the metabolism of liquids and all the different functions that help this metabolism of liquids and good circulation. In this case the Spleen is seen as joined together with the activities of the Lung and the Kidneys. You know the pathology that comes from this, when the Spleen is no longer able to metabolize and circulate liquids freely. If the Spleen is attacked you have the characteristic symptoms of a bloated, swollen abdomen, diarrhoea and tiredness, or you can even have emaciation, and every different illness to do with the retention of water. If there are phenomena of overheating then you can get the formation of *tan,* phlegm. All this depends on the location of the stagnation. Stagnation at the level of the skin and flesh gives oedema, but if it takes place in the intestines you have diarrhoea.

痰

The second great function of the Spleen is to participate in the production of Blood, and especially to have a particular effect on it, which is to retain and contain it. In other words, the Spleen is holding Blood in its form so that there is no erratic circulation, and it doesn't overflow out of the containing channels which are the *mai*. The quality of Blood partly depends on the juices that come from the Spleen, and the presence of the Spleen's function of Earth throughout the body at the level of the Blood gives it this ability to hold it in its correct form. Equally the connection between the Breaths and the Blood will come into play here, because we've said many times that the Spleen is the source of renewal for the Breaths, and the Blood can only move when it is animated by the Breaths. So in all these cases the Spleen maintains the Blood. The Chinese term gives the idea of presiding over the Blood like a chairman. For this reason, in practice if you are treating the Blood you also treat the Breaths. Many symptoms of haemorrhage can be linked with the Spleen, though obviously you have to take each case on its own. For example, one cause of irregularities in a woman's period is

脉

linked with the Spleen.

A third function is governing the four limbs. All external activities of movement are just a result of this function to transport, transform, to distribute nutrition and liquid elements and to be like a chairman for the Blood.

The Breaths of the Spleen also master ascending movement and that is in a complementary relation with the Breaths of the Stomach which circulate with a descending movement. This is essentially the exchange of Heaven and Earth, the ascending movement is the ascending of what is clear, pure and full of vitality, and the descending movement is the going down of what is unclear, impure and finally to be ejected. If these ascending and descending movements are disturbed, the clear *yang* Breaths can no longer be diffused and spread out, and Essences coming from Posterior Heaven can no longer return to the *zang* to be thesaurized. This ascending movement of the clear is also all the movement of circulation out to the extremities of the limbs, the skin and the hair on the skin, ie. out to the exterior. And the upward movement, the ascending of the clear, participates in the good maintenance and functioning of, for example, the orifices of the face, and the quality of Essences of the brain. We saw that the Stomach masters the descending movement, and with the Intestines governs all the doors and passages between the Stomach and Intestines and out to the exterior.

The Spleen likes dryness and fears dampness, and the Stomach likes humidity and fears dryness. We saw that this was because too much dampness blocks the movement of the *yang* of the Spleen, and too much dryness makes masceration and fermentation inside the Stomach impossible. As always we have this dual relationship between Stomach and Spleen in the well balanced humidity level within the organism.

Another special aspect is that the Spleen masters communication between the Heart and Kidneys, and that it is part of its function to be a turning point, a pivot. Sometimes it is thanks to the Spleen that communication between the Heart and the Kidneys is not lost, and it is sometimes to do with a blockage in the Spleen that communication between Heart and Kidneys is not properly adjusted.

Lastly, with the Breaths of the Stomach we saw their importance and how they have three main levels. One is simply the functioning of the Stomach, called the Breaths of the Stomach. The second is the level of the Spleen and Stomach functioning together which can also be called the Breaths of the Stomach maintaining a good balance between dampness and dryness, ascending and descending etc. The third level or meaning exists in quite a restricted sense, it is the role of the Stomach in governing whether you do or do not have an appetite.

The coating on the tongue gives indications for all the different *zang,* but it is particularly linked with the Stomach. The Stomach is also linked with all the aspects that the pulse presents, and with the aspects that the complexion gives, so you can see the different functions of the Stomach linked with the main diagnostic methods. The Nei Jing insists on the presence of the Stomach in the examination of the pulse, and you will know the importance of the Stomach in the coating on the tongue. Behind the complexion that you have will be the play between the Blood and the Breaths, and therefore here too the presence of the Stomach is felt.

APPENDIX

THE SPLEEN

The Spleen from the Nei Jing Jing Yi

絡表里

The Spleen is located in the middle of the abdomen; its meridian has a connecting, *luo,* and an internal / external, *biao li,* relation with the Stomach. The part of the body with which it is linked is the flesh; its orifice / opening is at the mouth.

運化精微清濁

Its functions are to master transportation and transformation, *yun hua,* to transmit and diffuse the *jing wei* which supply nutrition, to raise the clear, *qing,* and lower the unclear, *zhuo.* It is the source of the transformations that produce the Blood and its channeling; the five *zang* and the six *fu,* the four limbs and the one hundred bones rely on its nutrition.

氣統血痰後天之本

Its essential physiological functions are to enrich the *qi,* Breaths, to preside over the Blood , *tong xue,* to master the flesh and the four limbs, to transform phlegm, *tan,* and transform dampness....

Because of this the Spleen and Stomach were called by the ancients: the Root / Rooting of Posterior Heaven, *hou tian zhi ben.*

1. The Spleen masters transportation and transformation

運化精微水濕

The Spleen's function of transporting and transforming, *yun hua,* has two aspects: on the one hand the transportation and transformation of the *jing wei* drawn from the liquids and cereals, and on the other hand the transport and transformation of liquids and of dampness, *shui shi.*

The digestion of the liquids and cereals is the function of the Stomach;

124

精微

津液
脉　屬
絡

but the absorption of the *jing wei* from the liquids and cereals and their diffusion relies on the Spleen.

Spleen and Stomach each have their own area of activity in digestion as well as in the process of absorption and diffusion of the body fluids, *jin ye*. The Spleen meridian, the *tai yin* of the foot, is a *mai*, energy pathway, that crosses through the Stomach, has a dependent / belonging, *shu* relationship with the Spleen and a connecting, *luo*, relationship with the upper mouth of the oesophagus; in this way it can absorb the *jin ye* drawn from the liquids and cereals and transmit them to the three *yin* meridians.

表里

The Stomach is the granary, the storehouse for the absorption and nutrition of the five *zang* and the six *fu*. The Stomach meridian, the *yang ming* of the foot, is the *biao*, external, of the Spleen meridian, *tai yin*; the Spleen meridian is the *li*, internal, of the Stomach, *yang ming*. These two meridians have a *biao li*, internal / external, relationship and they are very closely and intimately linked.

津液

Thus, the *jin ye*, after being absorbed by the Spleen meridian, pass to the *yang ming* meridian through the free circulation maintained between them and are thus transmitted to the three *yang* meridians.

To summarize, the five *zang* and the six *fu*, even the four limbs and the one hundred bones, the layers of the skin, the muscles, the flesh... all the parts of the body must receive the influence of the Spleen meridian so that they can be nourished.

精微

In this way the Spleen masters the process of the transport and transformation of the *jing wei* from the liquids and cereals; and it is why, later on in medicine (that is to say after the Nei Jing), it was given the name: Root / Rooting of Posterior Heaven.

Regarding the digestion, transmission and diffusion of the *jin ye*, Spleen and Stomach, while each having their specific action, nonetheless work together and mutually influence each other.

土

The Spleen, being the *yin* of the element Earth, *tu,* is damp in nature and masters elevation / raising. The Stomach, being the *yang* of the element Earth, is dry in nature and masters lowering.

The dryness of the Stomach and the dampness of the Spleen act reciprocally and thus the food is well digested.

The nature of the Stomach is to govern lowering and thus the liquids and cereals can continue their descent. The nature of the Spleen is to govern raising and thus the *jin ye* can rely on it for transportation above.

Dryness and dampness, raising and lowering are opposites which complete each other. Thus the collaboration of the Spleen and Stomach brings about the perfect accomplishment of the whole process of transport and transformation of the liquids and cereals.

The Spleen does not merely transmit and circulate the *jin ye* from the Stomach to each part of the body to nourish the whole organism; it also transports and transforms the *qi,* Breaths, of the waters, *shui,* and the dampness, *shi,* of the whole body; it helps in the circulation and elimination of fluids, so maintaining the right balance in the body's liquid metabolism.

虚
浮腫

If the Spleen is empty, *xu,* it no longer has the strength needed for transporting, the liquids and dampness stagnate and this causes different kinds of oedema, *fu zhong,* congestion due to phlegm etc....

The Spleen's lack of strength in ensuring transportation is not the sole cause of the arrest and stagnation of liquids and dampness; but any stagnation of liquids and dampness has, on the other hand, a repercussion on the functions of the Spleen. It is commonly said that dampness hinders the Spleen - Earth. So, in Su Wen Chapter 23:

濕

The Spleen fears dampness, shi.

Digestion, absorption of nutrients, diffusion and distribution of the *jin ye,* are all the functions of the Spleen and Stomach; but the Small

126

Intestine, Large Intestine, Triple Heater and Bladder also have close connections with digestion, transportation of the *jin* and even the general liquid metabolism.

In the process of digestion, of absorption, of diffusion and evacuation, Spleen, Stomach, Small Intestine, Large Intestine, Triple Heater and Bladder have each their specific role; but if one performs its task badly, that has repercussions on the whole process of digestion, absorption and even evacuation.

2. The Spleen masters the flesh, its splendour is in the lips

The solid and liquid foods pass through the transportation and transformation, *yun hua,* as well as the absorption of the Spleen, so as to nourish the flesh. When this nutrition is carried out with sufficient strength, then the flesh is full and thriving.

If the Spleen is ill, this leads to a hampering of the proper functioning of digestion and absorption; the flesh loses what nourishes it and consequently it gradually gets thinner. So it is said in Su Wen Chapter 44:

The Spleen masters, zhu, the flesh, ji rou, of the body.

The fact that the Spleen masters the flesh is reflected in the lips. When the nutrition is not properly supplied, either because the Spleen is empty or ill for a long time, then this is shown in the colour and moistness of the lips and the mouth: they are yellow, dried up and dull. So, in Su Wen Chapter 10:

The reunion, he, of the Spleen is in the flesh. Its splendour, rong, is in the lips.

And Su Wen Chapter 9:

127

華 充 *Its flourishing aspect, hua, is at the four corners of the lips; the power of its fullness, chong, is in the flesh.*

Because of the links that exist between the Spleen on the one hand and the lips and mouth on the other, one can, by observing the aspects they present in their colour and moisture, deduce physiological and pathological changes that affect the Spleen and so prognose the evolution of the illness.

3. The Spleen masters the four limbs

For their activity the four limbs rely on the *yang* Breaths that come form the transformation of the solid and liquid foods. So, in Su Wen Chapter 30:

The four limbs are the root of all the yang

If the four limbs are the root of all the *yang,* how can the Spleen master the four limbs?

Su Wen Chapter 29 says:

When the Spleen is ill, the four limbs are out of use. How is this?
Qi Bo replied: The four limbs receive their Breaths, qi, from the Stomach, but these Breaths could not reach the meridians without the necessary support of the Spleen.

The upper and lower limbs rely, for their activation, on the *yang* Breaths that come from digestion; these Breaths certainly have their source in the transformation of solid and liquid food which occurs in the middle of the Stomach, but it is thanks to the transmission of the Spleen that the four limbs (and the meridians that run through them) can receive them. Thus the four limbs are indeed the root of all the *yang,* but they are dependent on that which is under the mastery of the Spleen, *tai yin,* Earth.

4. The Spleen presides over the Blood

精微

Not only does the Spleen ensure the functions of transporting and transforming, of diffusing the nourishing *jing wei*, of irrigating and nourishing the whole body, but it also has the function of containing the Blood. The Nan Jing Difficulty 42 says:

主裏
溫

The Spleen masters and envelopes, zhu guo, the Blood, warms, wen, the five zang.

Thus when the Breaths of the Spleen are vigorous and thriving they can envelope and protect the Blood, maintain the normality and regularity of the Blood circulation and ensure that it does not overflow, or leave its channels. If the functions of the Spleen are not well assured, this containing quality is lost and then the Blood overflows outside of the *mai* and all sorts of haemorrhages can be observed.

THE STOMACH

絡

The Stomach is located under the diaphragm; above it is linked to the oesophagus, below it communicates with the Small Intestine. Its meridian has a connecting, *luo,* relation with the Spleen.

The two doors and three cavities of the Stomach

賁門
幽門
上脘 下脘
中脘

The upper mouth of the Stomach is called *ben men,* door of precipitous rushing. The lower mouth of the Stomach is called *you men,* door of obscure depths. The region of *ben men* is called upper cavity, *shang wan,* and the region of *you men* is called lower cavity, *xia wan.* Between the upper and lower cavities is the middle cavity, *zhong wan.*

129

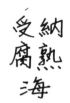

胃脘　These three parts together are called the cavities of the Stomach, *wei wan*.

The Stomach from the Zhong Yi Ji Qu Li Lun

The principal role of the Stomach is to receive the solid and liquid food and to initiate the process of digestion. To indicate that the Stomach masters the reception and introduction, *shou na*, the rotting (fermentation) and cooking, *fu shu*, of the liquids and cereals it is said that:

The Stomach is the Sea of liquids and cereals

The liquids and cereals that enter the Stomach pass through the first phase of digestion - the rotting and cooking - ensured by the Breaths of the Stomach; then the Small Intestine continues the process of digestion and absorption.

If the diet is not well regulated, either from eating too little or too much, eating irregularly, or if one eats inappropriately hot or cold food, all this has repercussions on the normal functions of the Stomach and that causes nausea, vomiting, hiccoughs, difficulties in digestion, stomach pains.... and other symptoms of countercurrent rising or of loss of harmony in the Breaths of the Stomach.

In traditional Chinese medicine the Breaths of the Stomach are particularly important:

When one has the Breaths of the Stomach one lives. If one no longer has the Breaths of the Stomach, one dies. When one has the Breaths of the Stomach, then one has the mechanics for life.

One must therefore be particularly vigilant, watch over the functions of the Stomach and pay close attention to them. One of the essential points in the therapeutic precepts of traditional Chinese medicine is to avoid at all costs taking longterm medicines that ruin the Breaths of the Stomach.

130

Su Wen Chapter 4

中央 土 — The central region, *zhong yang* is the Earth, *tu*

俞 脊 — The illness is in the Spleen and its *yu* on the spinal column, *ji*....

黄色 — The yellow aspect, *huang se,* of the Earth of the central region

入 通 脾 — It penetrates, *ru,* and communicates, *tong,* with the Spleen, *pi*

口 — It opens its orifice at the mouth, *kou*

藏 精 — It thesaurizes, *cang,* Essences, *jing,* in the Spleen

舌 本 — Thus its disturbance is located at the root of the tongue, *she ben*

甘 — Its taste is sweet, *gan*

土 — Its proper type is earth, *tu*

牛 — Its domestic animal is the ox, *niu*

稷 — Its cereal is millet, *ji*

肉 — Corresponding to the four seasons in the heights it is the planet Saturn, consequently the illness is seen in the flesh, *rou*

宮 — Its note is *gong,* (first on the pentatonic scale)

五 — Its number is five, *wu*

香 — Its odour is aromatic, *xiang*

中央　濕　The central region, *zhong yang,* produces dampness, *shi*

生　土　Dampness produces, *sheng,* Earth, *tu*

甘　　　Earth produces the sweet, *gan*

脾　　　Sweet produces the Spleen, *pi*

肉　　　Spleen produces the flesh, *rou*

　　　　Flesh produces the Lung

主　　　The Spleen is master, *zhu,* of the mouth

　　　　That which in Heaven makes dampness

地　土　On Earth, *di,* makes the earth, *tu*

　　　　In the body makes the flesh

藏　　　In the thesaurizations, *cang,* makes the Spleen

黃　　　In the coloured aspects makes yellow, *huang*

音　宮　In the notes, *yin,* makes the note *gong*

聲　歌　In the noises, *sheng,* makes singing, *ge*

變　動　In movements reacting to change, *bian dong,* makes eructations

竅　　　In the orifices, *qiao,* makes the mouth

味　In the Tastes, *wei,* makes the sweet

志　思　In the instances of will, *zhi,* makes meditative thought, *si*

Meditative thought injures the Spleen

勝　怒　That which victoriously balances out, *sheng,* meditative thought is anger, *nu*

Dampness injures the flesh

風　That which victoriously balances out dampness is wind, *feng*

Sweet injures the flesh

酸　That which victoriously balances out sweet is acid, *suan*.....

生　The Blood produces, *sheng,* the Spleen

Su Wen Chapter 8

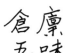 Spleen and Stomach are in charge of the storehouses and granaries, *cang lin;* the five tastes, *wu wei ,* stem from them.

133

Su Wen Chapter 9

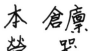

Spleen, Stomach, Large Intestine, Small Intestine, Triple Heater, Bladder: these are the root, *ben,* of the storehouses and granaries, *cang lin* , the dwelling place of nutrition, *ying.* Its name is utensil, *qi.*

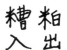

There is possibility for transformation giving residues and dregs, *zao po,* for the transmission of the Tastes as well as the entries and exits, *ru chu.*

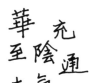

Its flourishing, *hua,* aspect is in the four whites of the lips, the power of its fullness, *chong,* is in the flesh; its taste is sweet, its colour yellow. Its category is extreme yin, *zhi yin* , and it is in free communication, *tong,* with the Breaths of the Earth, *tu qi.*

Su Wen Chapter 11

The Stomach is the Sea of liquids and cereals, the great gushing source of the six *fu.* The five Tastes enter the mouth and are stored in the Stomach to maintain, *yang,* the Breaths of the five *zang.*

Su Wen Chapter 18

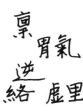

The normal Breaths of the well-balanced man (those that follow the norm of life) are received, *lin,* from the Stomach. The Stomach is the normal Breaths of the well-balanced man. When a man no longer has the Breaths of the Stomach, *wei qi,* then it is called counter current, *ni,* and this counter current is death.

....The great *luo* of the Stomach is called *xu li.* It crosses through the diaphragm and takes a connecting, *luo,* relation with the Lung. It comes out under the left breast. Its movement beats under the clothes.

They are the Ancestral Breaths of the *mai, mai zong qi.* When it overflows in fullness, whether there is panting, or whether it is frequent and interrupted: the illnesses are at the centre, *zhong.*

When it is knotted and transversal, there are accumulations, *ji.* If it is interrupted, *jue,* and no longer arrives, it is death. If under the breast its movement is echoed in the clothes (but too strongly): it is the Ancestral Breaths, *zong qi,* that flow out, *xie.*

Su Wen Chapter 19

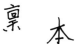

The five *zang* recieive, *lin*, the Breaths distributed from the Stomach. The Stomach is the root, *ben,* of the five *zang.*

Su Wen Chapter 22

The Spleen masters the long Summer. The *tai yin* and *yang ming* of the foot master the treatment. Its days are *wu* and *ji* (5th and 6th Heavenly Stems).

What affects the Spleen is dampness, *shi,* it is then urgent to eat bitter, *ku,* things to dry it out, *zao....*

The illnesses are in the Spleen: one is cured in Autumn. If one is not cured in Autumn, it intensifies in the Spring. If one does not die in Spring, it remains steady in Summer; one recovers in long Summer, *chiang xia.*

One should neither eat warm foods, nor eat too much nor remain on damp ground, nor wear soaking wet clothes.

甘 苦

The Spleen aspires to loosening, *huan* - temperance. One must quickly eat sweet things, *gan,* to loosen it (soften it). One uses bitter , *ku,* to disperse and sweet to tonify....

身重
善飢
肉痿 瘦

When the Spleen is ill, the body is heavy, *shen zhong.* One is easily hungry, *shan ji,* the flesh is flaccid, *rou wei,* the feet cannot receive (and walk correctly); when one walks one easily gets cramps, *chi,* one has pains in the lower part of the leg.

腹滿
腸鳴
飱瀉

In the case of emptiness the abdomen is congested, *fu man,* and the intestines gurgle *chang ming,* one has diarrhoea, *sun xie,* where food has not been digested: one takes (needles) the meridians concerned, *tai yin* and *yang ming,* as well as *shao yin,* bled....

大豆

The colour of the Spleen is yellow. It suits it to eat salty foods: large beans, *da dou,* pork, chestnuts, bean leaves (or peas). All that is salty.

Su Wen Chapter 52

市

The Spleen is the messenger, *shi;* the Stomach is the market, *shi.*

Ling Shu Chapter 17

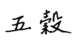

When the Breaths of the Spleen are in free communication with the mouth, the Spleen is in harmony and the mouth can distinguish the five cereals,*wu gu.*

136

Ling Shu Chapter 33

The Stomach is the Sea of liquids and cereals, *shui gu.* Its points of action at a distance, *shu,* are above at the Road of the Breaths, *qi jie,* Stomach 30, and below at *san li,* Stomach 36.

...Excess of the Sea of liquids and cereals: the abdomen is congested. Insufficiency of the Sea of liquids and cereals: one is hungry but when one eats one cannot accept the food.

Ling Shu Chapter 43

When the Breaths of the Spleen rise in power, *sheng,* one dreams of singing and music, *ge yue,* that the body is heavy and can no longer move....

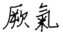

When the weakening Breaths , *jue qi* (introduction of perverse energies by countercurrent following on a deficiency of normal Breaths) are the hosts of the Spleen, in dreaming one sees mounds and hills and great marshes; one dreams that the house is ruined by wind and rain....When the weakening Breaths are the hosts of the Stomach, one dreams of drinking and eating.

SPLEEN/STOMACH PATHOLOGY

PRINCIPAL CAUSES OF DISEASE:

1. The Six Perverse Influences, *liu yin*

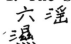

Dampness, *shi*, especially on the Spleen

Dryness, *zao,* especially on the Stomach

Cold, *han*, especially on the *yang* of the Spleen and Stomach

2. The Seven Emotions, *qi qing*

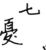

Overwhelming grief, *you,* Lung - Spleen relation

Meditative thought becoming preoccupation, *si*

Anger, *nu,* mastery of Liver-Wood over Spleen-Earth

3. Other Causes:

Diet - upset, excessive, insufficient, alcohol, too much cold food....

Tiredness - excessive tiredness, undermining the Original Breaths

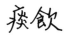

Phlegm and liquids, *tan yin,* which cause blockages

138

水氣　Breaths of waters, *shui qi:*　swellings, oedema

Parasites, especially coming from diet

Stagnation of unclear, linked here to dampness and setting off jaundice

Principal symptoms in these disorders:

- abnormal taste in the mouth

口喝　- dry mouth, *kou ke*

- one can eat and digest, but is easily hungry

嘈雜　- *cao za*

- one eats a lot but becomes thin

呃逆嘔吐　- hiccoughs and vomiting, *e ni ou tu*

噫氣噯腐　- burps, *yi qi,*　putrid eructations, *ai fu,*　acid regurgitation, *tan suan*

吞酸
　胃脘痛　- pains in the cavities of the Stomach, *wei wan tong*

腹痛　- pains in the abdomen, *fu tong*

腹瀉 便秘　- diarrhoea, *fu xie,*　and constipation, *bian mi*

- alteration in tongue coating

黃疸　- jaundice, *huang dan*

臌脹　- bloating, *gu zhang*

- toothache, swelling of the gums

痰飲 - phlegm and liquids, *tan yin*

帶下 - leucorrhea, *dai xia*

- collapse of the Central Breaths, leading especially to prolapse of organs

- haemorrhage and purpura

Spleen Patterns

脾氣虛 1. Emptiness of the Breaths of the Spleen, *pi qi xu*

脾陽虛 2. Emptiness of Spleen *yang, pi yang xu*

中氣下陷 3. The Central Breaths fall and collapse, *zhong qi xia xian*

脾不統血 4. The Spleen no longer presides over Blood, *pi bu tong xue*

寒濕困脾 5. Cold and damp hamper the Spleen, *han shi kun pi*

濕熱傷脾 6. Damp and heat injure the Spleen and Stomach, *shi re shang pi*

脾胃虛寒 7. Emptiness and cold of the Spleen and Stomach, *pi wei xu han*

脾虛水腫 8. Oedema through emptiness of the Spleen, *pi xu shui zhong*

Stomach Patterns

胃氣虛 1. Emptiness of the Breaths of the Stomach, *wei qi xu*

胃陰不足 2. Insufficient Stomach *yin, wei yin bu zu*

胃虛寒　3. Emptiness and cold of stomach, *wei xu han*

胃寒　4. Cold in the Stomach, *wei han*

胃熱　5. Heat in the Stomach, *wei re*

食滯胃脘 6. Blockage of food in the cavities of the Stomach, *shi zhi wei wan*

胃血瘀 7. Stagnation of Blood in the Stomach, *wei xue yu,* or

血瘀傷絡　Stagnation of Blood injures the network of communications, *xue yu shang luo*

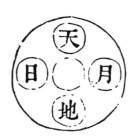